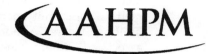

Hospice and Palliative Medicine

Core Curriculum and Review Syllabus

Editor
Ronald S. Schonwetter, MD, FACP

Coeditors
Wendy Hawke, MD
Carol F. Knight, EdM

American Academy of
Hospice and Palliative Medicine

KENDALL/HUNT PUBLISHING COMPANY
4050 Westmark Drive P.O. Box 1840 Dubuque, Iowa 52004-1840

The *Hospice and Palliative Medicine Core Curriculum and Review Syllabus* is sponsored by the American Academy of Hospice and Palliative Medicine. The publication is intended only to facilitate the free flow of information regarding hospice and palliative medicine within the medical community, particularly among clinicians involved in the care of patients with life-limiting illnesses. As additional research and clinical experience broaden current knowledge associated with this emerging field, continued changes in treatment and practice standards will be required.

No responsibility is assumed by the editors, authors, or the American Academy of Hospice and Palliative Medicine for any injury and/or damage to persons or property, as a matter of product liability, negligence, warranty, or otherwise, arising out of the use of application of any methods, products, instructions, or ideas contained herein. No guarantee, endorsement, or warranty of any kind, express or implied (including specifically no warrant of merchantability or of fitness for a particular purpose) is given by the Academy in connection with any information contained herein. Independent verification of any diagnosis, treatment, or drug use or dosage should be obtained. No test or procedure should be performed unless, in the judgment of an independent qualified physician, it is justified in light of the risk involved.

Inclusion of information in the publication does not constitute a guarantee, warranty, or endorsement by the American Academy of Hospice and Palliative Medicine of the quality, value, safety, effectiveness, or usefulness of any such product or of any claim made about such product by its manufacturer or an author.

Printing of this document was supported by an unrestricted educational grant from The Roxane Institute and Roxane Laboratories.

Citation: Schonwetter RS, Hawke W, Knight CF, eds. *Hospice and Palliative Medicine Core Curriculum and Review Syllabus*. American Academy of Hospice and Palliative Medicine. Dubuque, Iowa: Kendall/Hunt Publishing Company: 1999.

Cover image © 1998 PhotoDisc, Inc.

Copyright © 1999 by the American Academy of Hospice and Palliative Medicine
11250 Roger Bacon Drive Suite 8
Reston, Virginia 20190

ISBN 0-7872-5542-4

All rights reserved, including that of translation into other languages. No part of this publication may be reproduced or transmitted in any form or by any means, electronic or mechanical, including photocopying, recording, or any information storage and retrieval system, without permission in writing from the copyright holder.

Printed in U. S. A.

10 9 8 7 6 5 4 3 2 1

Contents

Acknowledgments

This curriculum and review syllabus was developed with help from many physicians and other professionals directly involved in the care of patients with life-limiting illnesses. The Academy's Board of Directors and the project director express their appreciation to the professionals who donated their time and expertise toward the development of this document. It is only with their ongoing dedication that the field of hospice and palliative medicine has become an integral component of mainstream medicine in the United States. The project director expresses his sincere gratitude to Gerald H. Holman, MD, who, more than ten years ago, developed a preliminary palliative medicine curriculum in conjunction with Paul Werner, MD and Carol Knight, EdM. Dr. Holman's continued work to refine the curriculum added immeasurably to the project. The project director also expresses his appreciation to Walter Forman, MD, President of the American Academy of Hospice and Palliative Medicine, for his ongoing support, leadership, and guidance.

The American Academy of Hospice and Palliative Medicine extends its gratitude to the following people for their contributions to the curriculum and review syllabus.

Project Director and Editor

Ronald S. Schonwetter, MD, FACP, CMD

Project Co-Editors

Wendy Hawke, MD
Carol F. Knight, EdM

Curriculum Authors

John W. Finn, MD
Medical Director
Hospice of Michigan
Southfield, Michigan

Walter B. Forman, MD, FACP, CMD
Professor
Department of Medicine
Division of Geriatrics
University of New Mexico Health Sciences
    Center
Albuquerque, New Mexico

Wendy Hawke, MD
Executive Vice-President of Administration
Director of Support Services and Palliative
    Care
Georgia Cancer Specialists
Atlanta, Georgia

David J. Hewitt, MD
Assistant Professor
Department of Neurology
The Emory Clinic
Emory University Medical Center
Atlanta, Georgia

Barry M. Kinzbrunner, MD, FACP
Vice-President/National Medical Director
Vitas Healthcare Corporation
Miami, Florida

Carol F. Knight, EdM
Knight Consultants
Austin, Texas

June Y. Leland, MD
Assistant Professor
Division of Geriatric Medicine
Department of Internal Medicine
University of South Florida College of
    Medicine
Director
Hospice and Community Medicine
James A. Haley VA Hospital
Tampa, Florida

Marcia Levetown, MD
Soros Faculty Scholar, Project on Death in
    America
Assistant Professor
Pediatrics, Internal Medicine, and Family
    Medicine
University of Texas Medical Branch
Pediatric Medical Director
Hospice Care Team and Houston Hospice
Galveston, Texas

David M. McGrew, MD
Medical Director
Hernando-Pasco Hospice
Hudson, Florida

Terry A. Melvin, MD
Clinical Instructor
Department of Internal Medicine & Family
    Medicine
University of Tennessee School of Medicine
Clinical Assistant Professor
Department of Family Medicine
East Tennessee State University
Medical Director
Hospice of Chattanooga
Chattanooga, Tennessee

Gary S. Reiter, MD, FACP
Assistant Professor of Medicine
University of Massachusetts Medical Center
Worcester, Massachusetts
Medical Director
River Valley HIV Clinic
Associate Medical Director
Hospice LifeCare of the VNS of Western
    Massachusetts
Holyoke, Massachusetts

Paul Rousseau, MD
Associate Chief of Staff for Geriatrics and
    Extended Care
VA Medical Center
Phoenix, Arizona

Charles G. Sasser, MD
Medical Director
Mercy Hospice of Horry County
Conway, South Carolina

Ronald S. Schonwetter, MD, FACP, CMD
Associate Professor
Division of Geriatric Medicine
Department of Internal Medicine
University of South Florida College of
    Medicine
Vice-President/Medical Director
LifePath Hospice
Tampa, Florida

John L. Shuster, Jr., MD
Soros Faculty Scholar, Project on Death in
    America
Associate Professor of Psychiatry
Associate Professor of Medicine
University of Alabama School of Medicine
Medical Director
University of Alabama in Birmingham
    Hospice
Birmingham, Alabama

Julia L. Smith, MD
Associate Professor
Oncology in Medicine
University of Rochester
Division Chief
Hematology/Oncology
Genesee Hospital
Medical Director
Hospice of Rochester
Rochester, New York

Mary B. Stegman, MD, FACP
Medical Director
Hope Hospice and Palliative Care
Fort Myers, Florida

Wendy M. Stein, MA, NHA, MD
Assistant Professor
Division of Geriatric Medicine
Department of Medicine
UCLA School of Medicine
Medical Director
Eisenberg Village
Jewish Home for the Aging
Reseda, California

Brad Stuart, MD
Medical Director
VNA & Hospice of Northern California
Santa Rosa, California

Charles F. von Gunten, MD, PhD
Assistant Professor of Medicine
Division of Hematology/Oncology
Department of Medicine
Northwestern University Medical School
Medical Director
Hospice and Palliative Care Program
Northwestern Memorial Hospital
Chicago, Illinois

Linda D. Wrede-Seaman, MD, FAAFP, FAEP
Medical Director
Providence Hospice of Yakima
Medical Director
Yakima Neighborhood Health Services
Yakima, Washington

Clifford L. Williams, MD
Medical Director
North Oaks Palliative Care Services
Hammond, Louisiana

Curriculum Review Panel

Carla S. Alexander, MD
Assistant Professor of Medicine
Divisions of Infectious Disease and
    Oncology
University of Maryland Medical System
Medical Director
Johns Hopkins Home Hospice
Baltimore, Maryland

David Barnard, PhD
University Professor of Humanities
Chairman, Department of Humanities
Penn State University College of Medicine
Hershey, Pennsylvania

Sandra L. Bertman, PhD
Professor, Humanities in Medicine
Director, Program of Medical Humanities
    and Palliative Care
University of Massachusetts Medical Center
Worcester, Massachusetts

Ira Byock, MD
Director, The Palliative Care Service
Research Professor of Philosophy
University of Montana
Missoula, Montana

Walter B. Forman, MD, FACP, CMD
Professor
Department of Medicine
Division of Geriatrics
University of New Mexico Health Sciences
   Center
Albuquerque, New Mexico

Michael E. Frederich, MD
Staff Physician
San Diego Hospice
San Diego, California

Gerald H. Holman, MD, FRCP, FAAP
Clinical Professor of Internal Medicine and
   Pediatrics
Assistant Clinical Professor of
   Pharmacology
Texas Tech School of Medicine
Vice-President of Medical Education
Crown of Texas Hospice
Amarillo, Texas

Jane Ingham, MB, BS, FRACP
Director
Palliative Care Program
Lombardi Cancer Center
Assistant Professor of Medicine
Department of Medicine
Georgetown University
Washington, DC

Gary A. Johanson, MD
Director of Palliative Care Services
Redwood Regional Medical Group
Medical Director
Spectrum Home Care and Hospice
Santa Rosa, California

Cheryl F. Jones, MD
Georgia Cancer Specialists
Assistant Professor
Division of Medical Oncology and Division
   of Palliative Medicine
Department of Family Practice
Mercer University School of Medicine
Macon, Georgia

Barry M. Kinzbrunner, MD, FACP
Vice-President/National Medical Director
Vitas Healthcare Corporation
Miami, Florida

June Y. Leland, MD
Assistant Professor
Division of Geriatric Medicine
Department of Internal Medicine
University of South Florida College of
   Medicine
Director
Hospice and Community Medicine
James A. Haley VA Hospital
Tampa, Florida

Michael H. Levy, MD, PhD
Director, Supportive Oncology Program
Fox Chase Cancer Center
Assistant Professor of Medicine
Temple University School of Medicine
Philadelphia, Pennsylvania

Jeanne G. Lewandowski, MD
Medical Director - Pediatrics
Bon Secours Hospital
Hospice of Michigan
Detroit, Michigan

David M. McGrew, MD
Medical Director
Hernando-Pasco Hospice
Hudson, Florida

Terry A. Melvin, MD
Clinical Instructor
Department of Internal Medicine & Family
   Medicine
University of Tennessee School of Medicine
Clinical Assistant Professor
Department of Family Medicine
East Tennessee State University
Medical Director
Hospice of Chattanooga
Chattanooga, Tennessee

Kathleen Murphy, MD
Geriatrician/Palliative Care Specialist
Marvin and Betty Dano Center
West Bloomfield, Michigan
Medical Director
Hospice of Michigan
Southfield, Michigan

Paul Rousseau, MD
Associate Chief of Staff for Geriatrics and
    Extended Care
VA Medical Center
Phoenix, Arizona

Porter Storey, MD, FACP
Clinical Associate Professor of Medicine
Assistant Professor of Family Medicine
Baylor College of Medicine
Consultant in Neuro-Oncology
Adjunct Assistant Professor of Medicine
University of Texas M.D. Anderson Cancer
    Center
Medical Director
The Hospice at the Texas Medical Center
Houston, Texas

Martha L. Twaddle, MD
Assistant Professor of Clinical Medicine
Northwestern University School of
    Medicine
Senior Attending in Internal Medicine
Evanston Hospital
Faculty in Palliative Medicine
Lurie Cancer Center
Northwestern University
Medical Director
Hospice of the North Shore
Evanston, Illinois

Charles F. von Gunten, MD, PhD
Assistant Professor of Medicine
Division of Hematology/Oncology
Department of Medicine
Northwestern University Medical School
Medical Director
Hospice and Palliative Care Program
Northwestern Memorial Hospital
Chicago, Illinois

David E. Weissman, MD
Professor of Medicine
Director
Palliative Care Program
Medical College of Wisconsin
Milwaukee, Wisconsin

David I. Wollner, MD
Assistant Professor of Medicine
Albert Einstein College of Medicine
Attending Physician
Department of Pain Medicine and Palliative
    Care
Beth Israel Medical Center
New York, New York

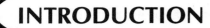

INTRODUCTION

Introduction to Hospice and Palliative Medical Education

Hospice and Palliative Medical Education

Despite increased societal concern about end-of-life issues, there is no clear indication that care for most patients with life-limiting illnesses has improved significantly. Increased attention has been given to hospice and palliative medical education; however, in practice, the majority of physicians, medical students, and residents receive sporadic and unstructured training in the principles and practice of caring for patients with advanced, life-limiting illnesses.

In the United States, medical conferences devote limited space to palliative medicine and research, and only five of 126 medical schools surveyed in 1994 offered a separate required course on death and dying. Only 26 percent of residency programs offer a specific course on end-of-life care. Many physicians, medical students, and residents acknowledge a lack of skill and confidence in the area of palliative medicine, and desire more education and training on symptom control and the management of psychosocial and spiritual concerns.

In its report on end-of-life care, the Institute of Medicine (IOM) suggests the following:

- Undergraduate, graduate, and continuing education do not sufficiently prepare physicians to provide effective care for dying patients;

- Physicians have a special responsibility for educating themselves and others about the identification and management of the last phases of terminal illness;
- Despite the availability of effective options for relieving most pain, too many dying people suffer needlessly from serious pain and other distressing symptoms that clinicians could prevent or relieve with existing knowledge and therapies;
- Due to errors of omission and commission, many dying patients suffer needlessly at the end of life; both under-treatment and over-treatment often prolong suffering.

To improve education and training on end-of-life care, the Institute of Medicine, the American Medical Association, the American Board of Internal Medicine, and other organizations recommend the following:

- Palliative care should become, if not a medical specialty, at least a defined area of expertise, education, and research;
- Practitioners must hold themselves and their colleagues responsible for using existing knowledge and available interventions to assess, prevent, and relieve physical and emotional distress;
- Educators and other health professionals should initiate changes in undergraduate, graduate, and continuing education to ensure practitioners have appropriate attitudes, knowledge, and skills to care for dying patients;

- Medical schools and residency programs should provide comprehensive structured training on end-of-life care;
- Educational materials should be developed which acknowledge the reality that people die and that continued caring is the only humane option;
- Readily available, practical formats should be developed for transmitting current information about end-of-life care to medical residents, residents, and attending physicians.

Curriculum Goals and Objectives

This curriculum and review syllabus is based on the current substantial body of knowledge comprising hospice and palliative medicine. It is the first core curriculum and review syllabus on hospice and palliative medicine in the United States developed primarily by palliative medicine physicians. The curriculum focuses on the following elements identified by the Institute of Medicine as essential for effective end-of-life care:

- Effective techniques for assessing and controlling pain and other distressing symptoms;
- Alleviating death-related psychological and spiritual distress;
- Assessing and managing complicated grief reactions;
- Communicating effectively with patients and family members;
- Making ethical decisions;
- Participating on interdisciplinary teams;
- Cultivating empathy and sensitivity to religious, ethnic, cultural, and other differences.

The goal of the curriculum is to develop physicians and other health care professionals who are knowledgeable scientists and competent, compassionate practitioners of hospice and palliative medicine. Physicians should demonstrate abilities in the following areas:

the provision of appropriate palliative interventions for patients with life-limiting illnesses; effective interactions with dying patients and their families; and full collaboration with other healthcare professionals to ensure patients receive comprehensive care to alleviate their suffering.

The primary objectives of the curriculum and review syllabus are to describe the core elements of hospice and palliative medicine, to reinforce the development of appropriate attitudes toward patients with life-limiting illnesses, to summarize the requisite body of knowledge, and to describe the skills necessary for the effective practice of hospice and palliative medicine.

Recognizing the variety of educational settings and differences among physicians in terms of knowledge, training, experience, and time for continuing education, the curriculum is designed to be as flexible as possible. It consists of a series of modules, each of which includes a brief narrative summary of a specific topic, objectives, and a list of references. As recommended by the World Health Organization, the curriculum's objectives focus on three interrelated domains of palliative medicine education: (1) attitudes, values, and behaviors; (2) knowledge base; and (3) skills.

The curriculum and review syllabus is not meant to be a comprehensive textbook on palliative medicine; instead it is targeted to medical educators and practicing physicians interested in advancing their knowledge and skills in palliative medicine. The review syllabus provides a general overview of the practice of hospice and palliative medicine, and the list of topics is not exhaustive. The syllabus attempts to provide current information; however, the Academy recognizes that the field is continuing to evolve—even its definition is subject to change. New advances in knowledge, standards, and approaches to care will be included in future editions. The curriculum should be amended as appropriate when designing educational experiences to meet the needs of specific learners, that is, medical students; residents in internal medicine, oncology, geriatrics, and family practice; and other practicing physicians.

The style and format of instruction vary considerably among medical schools. Some schools designate specific teaching blocks for palliative medicine, but in most cases, the principles and practice of palliative medicine are incorporated in other curriculum blocks. To improve the teaching of palliative medicine in medical school settings, Scott and MacDonald suggest several strategies, including the following:

- Concentrate on defining the goals and integrating the concepts of palliative medicine throughout the current curriculum instead of focusing solely on increasing the number of dedicated courses on palliative medicine;
- Help colleagues from other disciplines incorporate the principles and practice of palliative medicine in teaching, and provide them with case studies and other teaching materials for use in didactic courses, small-group learning, and other experiences;
- Involve as role models faculty whose behavior illustrates the principles of palliative medicine;
- Demonstrate the principles of palliative medicine by including other members of an interdisciplinary team in teaching, for example, nurses, social workers, and chaplains;
- Change students' attitudes and behavior and improve learning by providing "hands-on" experiences, for example, guided contact with patients and families ;
- Incorporate well-designed small-group teaching, seminars, and clinical rotations;
- Use educational manuals, videos, computerized instruction, and other informational aids to enhance learning;
- Include questions about the principles and practice of palliative medicine in student examinations.

Methods for Teaching Hospice and Palliative Medicine

In general, effective teaching methods incorporate the following:

- Experiential, interactive, educational experiences
- Faculty collaboration
- Presentation of lectures and seminars after students have interacted personally with patients and listened to their needs and concerns
- Experiences that increase students' awareness of their preconceived notions about dying and fears of interacting with dying patients, the importance of establishing compassionate doctor/patient relationships, and a dying patient's identity as a real person living with a real family, often in difficult circumstances

Depending on the setting and the needs of learners, the following strategies can be effective for teaching the principles and practice of hospice and palliative medicine:

- Reading and lectures
- Case studies
- Computer-assisted learning
- Attending interdisciplinary conferences
- Bedside teaching, including home visits
- Experiential learning, for example, small group projects, small group discussions, role plays, and journaling

Examples of innovative teaching methods include the following:

- Interaction with patients with life-limiting illnesses and their family members, often via hospice and palliative medicine rotations and visits to patients' homes with members of the interdisciplinary team
- Small group study of the impact of terminal illness and death on an entire family

system, especially with regard to cultural and religious practices
- Role-playing communication techniques for sharing bad news and discussing psychosocial and spiritual concerns
- Following patients with advanced illnesses throughout the illness trajectory
- Observing palliative medicine consultations

- Using patient and clinical narratives, literature, and structured opportunities for personal reflection
- Using standardized, simulated patients

Key references are included at the end of the curriculum to assist those desiring an overview of hospice and palliative medicine.

References

1. Billings JA, Block S. Palliative care in undergraduate medical education: status report and future directions. *JAMA*. 1997;278(9):733-738.
2. Blank LL. Defining clinical competence and strategies for evaluation. In: *Caring for the Dying: Identification and Promotion of Physician Competency*. Philadelphia, Pa: American Board of Internal Medicine; 1996:41-44.
3. Bruera E. Research in symptoms other than pain. In: Doyle D, Hanks GWC, MacDonald N, eds. *Oxford Textbook of Palliative Medicine*. New York: Oxford University Press; 1993:87-92.
4. Byock IR. The nature of suffering and the nature of opportunity at the end of life. *Clin Geriatric Med*. 1996;12(2):237-252.
5. Canadian Committee on Palliative Care Education. *The Canadian Palliative Care Curriculum*. 1991.
6. *Cancer Pain Relief and Palliative Care: Technical Report Series 804*. Geneva: World Health Organization; 1990.
7. Cassel CK. Overview on attitudes of physicians toward caring for the dying patient. In: *Caring for the Dying: Identification and Promotion of Physician Competency*. Philadelphia, Pa: American Board of Internal Medicine; 1996:1-4.
8. Cassell EJ. *The Nature of Suffering and the Goals of Medicine*. New York: Oxford University Press; 1991.
9. Clark H. Common experiences of physicians and relevant teaching strategies. In: *Caring for the Dying: Identification and Promotion of Physician Competency*. Philadelphia, Pa: American Board of Internal Medicine; 1996:33-38.
10. Cox J. Caring for the dying.: reflections of a medical student. *CMAJ*. 1987;136:577-579.
11. Field MJ, Cassel CK, eds. *Approaching Death: Improving Care at the End of Life*. Report by the Committee on Care at the End of Life. Institute of Medicine. Washington, D.C.: National Academy Press; 1997.
12. Foley KM. Palliative medicine, pain control, and symptom assessment. In: *Caring for the Dying: Identification and Promotion of Physician Competency*. Philadelphia, Pa: American Board of Internal Medicine. 1996;11-26.
13. Hill TP. Treating the dying patient: the challenge for medical education. *Arch Intern Med*. 1995;155:1265-1269.
14. Knight, CF, Knight PF, Gellula M, Holman GH. Training our future physicians: a hospice rotation for medical students. *Am J Hospice Palliat Care*. 1992; 9(1):23-28.
15. Liaison Committee on Medical Education 1992-1993 Annual Medical School Questionnaire, Part II. Reported by: Council on Scientific Affairs, American Medical Association. Good care of the dying patient. *JAMA*. 1996;275(6):474-478.
16. Martinez JM, Neely KJ, Preodor ME, Twaddle M, von Gunten C. *Teaching Hospice/Palliative Care*. Presented at the 9th Annual Assembly of the American Academy of Hospice and Palliative Medicine. Chicago, Illinois: June 25-28, 1997.
17. Martini CJM. Grenholm G. Institutional responsibility in graduate medical education and highlights of historical data. *JAMA*. 1993;270:1053-1060.

18. Schechter, GP. Professionalism in providing end-of-life patient care. In: *Caring for the Dying: Identification and Promotion of Physician Competency*. American Board of Internal Medicine. 1996:5-7.

19. Schonwetter RS, ed. *Clinics in Geriatric Medicine*. Care of the Terminally Ill Patient. Philadelphia: WB Saunders: 1996;12(2):237-433.

20. Schonwetter RS, Robinson BE. Teaching palliative care to medical students as part of a fourth year geriatric elective. *J Am Geriatr Soc*. 1992;40(10):SA87.

21. Schonwetter RS, Robinson BE. Educational objectives for medical training in the care of the terminally ill. *Acad Med*. 1994;69(8):688-690.

22. Scott JF, MacDonald N. Education in palliative medicine. In: Doyle D, Hanks GWC, MacDonald N, eds. *Oxford Textbook of Palliative Medicine*. New York: Oxford University Press; 1993:761-781.

23. *Standards of a Hospice Program of Care*. Arlington, Va: National Hospice Organization; 1993.

24. von Gunten CF, Von Roenn JH. Barriers to pain control: ethics & knowledge. *J Palliat Care*. 1994;10:52-54.

25. von Gunten CF, Von Roenn JH, Gradishar W, Weitzman S. Hospice/palliative medicine rotation for fellows training in hematology/oncology. *J Cancer Edu*. 1995;10:200-203.

26. von Gunten CF, Von Roenn JH, Neely KJ, Martinez J, Weitzman S. Hospice and palliative care: attitudes and practices of the physician faculty of an academic hospital. *Am J Hospice Palliat Care*. 1995;12:38-42.

27. Weissman DE. Pre-clinical palliative medicine education at the Medical College of Wisconsin. *J Cancer Educ*. 1993;8:191-195.

28. Weissman DE. Consultation in palliative medicine. *Arch Intern Med*. 1997;157:733-737.

29. Working Party of the Association for Palliative Medicine. *Palliative Medicine Curriculum*. Southampton, Hampshire, United Kingdom: Association for Palliative Medicine of Great Britain and Ireland; 1991.

Hospice and Palliative Medicine: Philosophy, History, and Standards of Care

Hospice and Palliative Medicine

During the early stages of a serious illness, treatment is generally aggressive and the goal of care is cure or remission of disease. As the illness progresses, the burdens of traditional medical therapies may begin to outweigh their benefits. The patient and/or physician may then change the goals of care. The transition period from traditional curative care to palliative care can be one of the most difficult phases of caring for patients with life-limiting illnesses. Nevertheless, when cure is not possible, treatment goals appropriately change from prolonging life to controlling symptoms and maximizing quality of life so patients remain as comfortable as possible throughout the entire illness trajectory.

Palliative medicine is the study and management of patients with active, progressive, far advanced disease for whom the prognosis is limited and the focus of care is quality of life. The discipline recognizes the multidimensional nature of suffering, responds with care that addresses all dimensions of suffering, and communicates in language that conveys mutuality, respect, and interdependence.

Hospice and palliative medicine emphasize advanced planning and ongoing care and support, rather than crisis intervention and episodic involvement by healthcare professionals. Physicians practicing hospice and palliative medicine often provide care in home settings, which not only allows patients and families to remain in control of their care and surroundings but also offers opportunities to educate medical students about non-institutional approaches to symptom management.

Although hospice and palliative medicine focus on the management of pain and non-pain symptoms (e.g., dyspnea, anorexia, chronic fatigue, nausea, constipation, anxiety, weakness, and depression), emphasis is placed on relieving all aspects of suffering. Promoting psychosocial and spiritual growth and development is one of the ultimate goals of hospice and palliative care. With skilled clinical interventions and emotional and spiritual support from family members and professional caregivers, patients are more likely to experience a sense of increased satisfaction, completion, and personal growth as their lives draw to a close.

The World Health Organization (WHO) estimates that anticancer treatments and curative therapies account for approximately 80 percent of the allocation of cancer resources in developed countries, with relief of cancer pain and palliative therapies receiving only 20 percent of the resources. The WHO suggests that curative and palliative care are not mutually exclusive, and recommends reallocating resources to support symptom management and whole-person care throughout the illness continuum. Because resources are limited and few (if any) curative treatments are available for much of the world's population, the WHO proposes that palliative care begin at diagnosis and gradually become an increasing component of care until death occurs.

Palliative treatments are treatments and interventions that enhance comfort and improve a patient's quality of life. No specific therapy is excluded from consideration. The test of a palliative treatment lies in agreement by the physician, patient, primary caregiver, and interdisciplinary team that a treatment's expected outcome is relief from distressing symptoms and enhanced quality of life. The decision to intervene with an active palliative treatment is based on the treatment's ability to meet stated goals, rather than its effect on the underlying disease. In addition to traditional pharmacologic methods of symptom control, adjuvant complementary therapies may include music therapy, acupuncture, aromatherapy, meditation, special diets, and many other therapies.

Radiation, chemotherapy, surgery, and other aggressive palliative measures have appropriate uses in hospice and palliative medicine, as long as the goal of therapy is symptom relief, and the benefits of treatment outweigh the burdens. In any case, patients are continually assessed, and all treatment options are explored and evaluated within the context of the patient's wishes and the goals of care.

Philosophy of Palliative Care and Hospice Care

The World Health Organization (WHO) defined palliative care as the active total care of patients whose diseases are not responsive to curative treatment. Compassionate symptom control is paramount, and includes the alleviation of symptoms, whether they are physical, psychological, emotional, social, or spiritual. Equal emphasis is placed on providing emotional support for patients and families as they cope with the multiple losses associated with terminal illness.

Total palliative care usually involves an interdisciplinary team of healthcare professionals who provide coordinated medical, nursing, psychosocial, and spiritual care services. The goal of palliative care is to achieve the best possible quality of life for patients and their families, which requires expert clinical intervention and compassionate support for patients and their families as they search for a sense of physical, psychological, social, and spiritual well-being. Many aspects of palliative care are also applicable early in the course of an illness, in conjunction with disease-specific treatment.

The term *palliative care* originally referred to the care of patients with terminal illnesses, but now refers to the care of patients with life-limiting illnesses, whether or not they are imminently dying. Philosophically, the relief of suffering and the enhancement of a patient's quality of life are the primary objectives of both palliative care and hospice care. Although general hospice and palliative care approaches are similar and may be provided along the continuum of care for patients with life-limiting illnesses, hospice care is generally provided during the latter segments of the continuum.

Historical Perspectives

The earliest recorded hospice was established by a Christian religious order in Rome in 475 CE. There, weary travelers, pilgrims from Africa, and the dying could find comfort, refuge, and spiritual renewal. During the Middle Ages, Christian religious orders established networks of hospices across Europe.

Hospice programs developed in response to the unmet physical, social, emotional, and spiritual needs of terminally ill patients. Currently, many hospice programs in the United States are responding to the challenges of cultural and religious diversity by developing staff training programs designed to improve the care of patients from all faith traditions.

Great Britain and Ireland

The modern hospice movement began when Sister Mary Aikenhead founded the Irish Sisters of Charity, and later opened Our Lady's Hospice for the Dying in Dublin in 1879. In 1905, the Irish Sisters opened St. Joseph's Hospice for the Dying in Hackney. It was there that Cicely Saunders, a remarkable hospice pioneer, later developed the principles of modern hospice and palliative medicine, for example, management of pain using opioid analgesics administered around-the-clock, emphasis on relieving the multi-faceted components of total pain, and an interdisciplinary approach to comprehensive and compassionate care.

Dr. Saunders trained as a nurse, a social worker, and a physician. In 1967, she opened St. Christopher's Hospice in Sydenham, London, which continues to serve as one of the world's preeminent hospice programs, focusing on patient care, education, research, and innovation. Throughout her career, Dr. Saunders emphasized the importance of diligent application of the science of hospice and palliative medicine and the equal importance of emotional and spiritual care. In Great Britain and Ireland, hospice care is a well-recognized and integrated component of the healthcare system. It is institutionally based, emphasizing free-standing inpatient facilities, hospital support teams, and complementary home care services. In 1987, palliative medicine was recognized as a specialty by the Royal College of Medicine.

The United States

In the United States, hospice was born as an alternative to the increasing medicalization and institutionalization of death. In an era of unlimited hospitalization and routine application of technology, most patients died in institutions while receiving intravenous fluids, nutritional support, resuscitation, and other invasive and often futile interventions.

The earliest hospice programs relied on professional and nonprofessional caregivers who offered their assistance on a volunteer basis and provided support for people who wished to die in the comfort of their own homes, with their families present and with minimal medical intrusion. In general, the medical community reacted negatively to the hospice approach to dying, which they viewed as being opposed to medical science and patient survival. However, as patients continued to seek hospice care, the number of hospice programs grew, which gained the attention of national healthcare policy makers.

Over the years, hospice care has grown from an alternative healthcare movement to an established component of the healthcare system. The first inpatient hospice program opened in New Haven, Connecticut in 1974. By 1996 approximately 450,000 patients were served by 2,700 hospice programs.

Medicare Hospice Benefit

Based on the findings of the National Hospice Study, the 1982 Tax Equity and Fiscal Responsibility Act (TEFRA) established the Medicare Hospice Benefit, which became effective on November 1, 1983. The Medicare Hospice Benefit established conditions of participation and defined terminality, which has had profound effects on the care of dying people in the United States.

Medicare-certified hospice programs must provide comprehensive palliative care for terminally ill patients and supportive services to their families and significant others. Physical, social, spiritual, and emotional care must be provided by an interdisciplinary team of skilled healthcare professionals (including a physician), who focus on relieving the patient's and family's suffering during the later stages of illness, during the dying process, and during the family's bereavement for at least 12 months after the patient's death.

For purposes of the Medicare Hospice Benefit, terminally ill patients are defined as having a prognosis of six months or less, if the disease runs its normal course.

Standards of Care

Role of Hospice Programs

Hospice programs provide comprehensive palliative care to terminally ill patients and supportive services to their families and significant others, 24 hours a day, seven days a week, in both home and facility-based settings. With physician oversight, physical, social, spiritual, and emotional care are provided during the later stages of illness, during the dying process, and during bereavement, by an interdisciplinary team consisting of patients/families, professionals, and volunteers.

The hospice philosophy of care views dying as a natural part of the life cycle. Practitioners seek neither to hasten nor postpone death, but instead to provide comfort and supportive care while a patient's life-limiting illness runs its natural course. In hospice and palliative care, primary emphasis is not on death and dying, but on living each day fully until death occurs. In addition to aggressive symptom management, supportive hospice and palliative care interventions can help patients achieve a renewed and redefined sense of hope, worthiness, meaning, purpose, and completion as their lives draw to a close.

Unit of Care

In hospice and palliative care, the patient and family comprise the unit of care. The patient is viewed not as a disease, but as a person who is a member of an entire family system. Hospice programs emphasize empowerment of patients and families. Surveys generally reveal high family satisfaction with hospice services, due in part to the inclusion of family members in decision making and the ongoing emotional support provided to family

members throughout the patient's illness and during the bereavement period.

Hospice team members recognize the family's need for information, for help with practical matters, for assistance with decision making, and for ongoing discussions of their concerns. Initial and ongoing evaluations help patients and families define their individual needs, set realistic goals, and make appropriate treatment choices. When patients are free from physical distress and when their psychosocial and spiritual concerns have been addressed, both the patient and family are more likely to experience a comfortable ending of the patient's life. Often during the dying process, patients and family members express love and forgiveness and, in cases of prior estrangement, may achieve some measure of reconciliation.

Interdisciplinary Team

Hospice care focuses on relieving physical pain, as well as on alleviating suffering experienced by terminally ill patients and their family members. Effective interventions require the skills and resources of an entire team of healthcare professionals. The interdisciplinary team provides support and guidance for patients and families as they confront common challenges associated with dying. The team's combined professional and personal perspectives are much more likely to meet the complex needs of dying patients and their families. Team members include physicians, nurses, home health aides, social workers, clergy, volunteers, and other specialized healthcare professionals as needed.

Nurses coordinate the patient's care, communicate with attending physicians and other members of the team, assess the patient's and family's needs, and supervise care in the patient's home and other settings. Home health aides bathe patients, assist with activities of daily living, offer comfort measures, and report changes in the patient's or family's condition to a nurse. Social workers help patients and families access community resources and provide counseling for death-related issues, including communication problems, anticipatory grief, and bereavement issues. Clergy address spiritual and religious issues, coordinate and/or provide spiritual and religious interventions, and offer spiritual support for patient and family members. Volunteers assist patients in a multitude of ways, for example, companionship, grocery shopping, preparing light meals, mowing lawns, and the like.

Physicians practicing in palliative and hospice care settings collaborate with all members of the interdisciplinary team to ensure that all aspects of suffering are addressed, that is, physical, social, spiritual, and psychological distress. Physicians caring for terminally ill patients outside hospice settings should develop their own informal teams to ensure they adequately meet the complex needs of both patients with life-limiting illnesses and the patient's family members.

Barriers to Hospice and Palliative Care

Despite a rapid increase in the number of hospice programs, only 20 percent of the total number of patients eligible for the Medicare Hospice Benefit receive hospice care. Barriers to hospice care include late referrals and difficulties with prognosis. Terminally ill patients often are referred for hospice care late in the course of their disease—median survival was 36 days in 1990 and is significantly less today.

Late referrals are due partly to physician's attitudes about death. Physicians may view a patient's death as a medical and personal failure. When curative goals are no longer

appropriate, physicians may believe they have nothing left to offer. Instead of communicating with patients and families about revised goals of treatment and palliative care, they may distance themselves from patients because they are uncomfortable talking about death-related issues. However, earlier referrals allow patients and families to receive greater benefit from hospice services, for which patients and families are generally grateful.

Prognosis-related issues also serve as barriers to hospice care. Accurately predicting prognosis is difficult, particularly when a patient has a non-cancer disease. In recent years, as the percentage of non-cancer patients being served by hospices has increased to 40 percent, accurate prognosis is even more important. To help physicians assess a patient's appropriateness for hospice care and eligibility for the Medicare Hospice Benefit, the National Hospice Organization published the second edition of the *Medical Guidelines for Determining Prognosis in Selected Non-Cancer Diseases.*

Recent societal emphasis on improving the quality of life of patients with advanced disease has had a significant impact on the care of dying patients, and has fostered general acceptance of the concept of palliative care, instead of the continued provision of futile, life-prolonging interventions.

Improved patient access to comprehensive hospice and palliative services must be achieved if palliative care is to serve as an alternative to physician-assisted suicide. Organizations must provide comprehensive, skilled care for all patients with life-limiting illnesses and must establish innovative programs with hospitals, medical schools, and insurers to reduce barriers to much-needed care.

Objectives

Attitudes/Behaviors

1. Discuss the continuum from traditional curative care to palliative care for patients with life-limiting illnesses.

2. Discuss the role of hospice and palliative care in the continuum of care for patients with life-limiting illnesses.

3. Defend each patient's individual needs during the course of a life-limiting illness.

4. Discuss the integration of hospice care into the healthcare system in the United States.

5. Describe the reasons for the emergence of hospice and palliative care in the United States.

6. Defend the concept of whole-person care in hospice and palliative care.

7. Discuss the importance of viewing the patient and family as the unit of care.

8. Describe the characteristics of palliative interventions.

9. Discuss the physician's role when caring for chronically and terminally ill patients.

10. Defend the concept of palliation as an appropriate treatment goal for patients with a life-limiting illness.

11. Describe the multifactorial needs of patients with life-limiting illnesses.

12. Explain why hospice and palliative care are not defined solely by the Medicare Hospice Benefit.

13. Describe the comprehensive goals of palliative care.

14. Discuss the need for an interdisciplinary approach to caring for patients with life-limiting illnesses.

15. Describe the difficulties associated with prognostication and their effects on referring patients for hospice and palliative care.

16. Discuss multiple contributors to suffering, e.g., physical, psychosocial, emotional, and spiritual factors.

17. Defend the need for adequate access to hospice and palliative care services for patients with life-limiting illnesses.

18. Describe the need for open, honest, compassionate communication with terminally ill patients and their family members.

19. Discuss dying as a natural part of the life cycle.

20. Honor a patient's wishes when making medical decisions about treatments and the goals of care.

Knowledge

1. Describe the origins of hospice and palliative care both nationally and internationally.

2. Discuss the major goals and concepts of the hospice and palliative medicine approach to caring for patients with life-limiting illnesses.

3. Describe common conditions that result in chronic and terminal illness, including their usual presentations and progression.

4. Describe the concept of *total pain*.

5. Discuss common symptoms experienced by terminally ill patients near the end of life.

6. Describe eligibility requirements for the Medicare Hospice Benefit.

7. Describe the distinction between determining a patient's eligibility for admission to a hospice program and certifying a patient as eligible for the Medicare Hospice Benefit.

8. Discuss the roles of individual members of a hospice interdisciplinary care team.

9. Describe the development of the Medicare Hospice Benefit.

10. Describe the National Hospice Organization's guidelines for determining prognosis in non-cancer patients.

11. Discuss the role of the physician as a member of a hospice and palliative care interdisciplinary team.

12. Describe multiple barriers to hospice and palliative care services.

13. Discuss the World Health Organization's recommendations for changes in the allocation of resources for cancer treatment.

Skills

1. Use the National Hospice Organization's *Medical Guidelines for Determining Prognosis in Selected Non-Cancer Disease* to determine as accurately as possible the prognosis of a patient with a life-limiting illness.

2. Participate as an effective member of an interdisciplinary team when caring for terminally ill patients and their family members.

3. Discuss palliative treatment options with terminally ill patients and their families, and consider the potential benefits and burdens of each option.

4. Communicate effectively about death-related issues with patients, families, and other health professionals.

5. Respond appropriately to patients who ask for assistance with suicide.

6. Make appropriate referrals for problems that cannot be handled by the physician.

7. Practice hospice and palliative medicine in a variety of settings, e.g., the patient's home, a nursing facility, an acute care setting, and a hospice or palliative care inpatient unit.

8. Assist patients and families with the transition from traditional curative care to palliative care.

9. Apply appropriate concepts of hospice and palliative medicine to patient care throughout the illness trajectory.

10. Consider the patient's values, medical condition, and goals of treatment when making recommendations about palliative interventions.

11. Assess the presence of total pain in a terminally ill patient, considering physical, emotional, social, and spiritual factors contributing to suffering.

References

1. Berry ZS, Lynn J. Hospice medicine. *JAMA*. 1993;270:221-223.
2. Bulkin W, Lukashok H. Rx for dying: the case for hospice. *N Engl J Med*. 1988;318:376-378.
3. Byock IR. The nature of suffering and the nature of opportunity at the end of life. *Clin Geriatric Med*. 1996;12(2):237-252.
4. Callahan D. *The Troubled Dream of Life; In Search of a Peaceful Death*. Portland, Ore: Touchstone Press; 1996.
5. *Cancer Pain Relief and Palliative Care: Report of a WHO Expert Committee*. Geneva, Switzerland: World Health Organization Technical Report Series. 1990;804.
6. Christakis N, Escarese J. Survival of Medicare patients after enrollment in hospice programs. *N Engl J Med*. 1996;335:172-8.
7. Cleeland CS, Gonin R, Hatfield AK, et. al. Pain and its treatment in outpatients with metastatic cancer. *N Engl J Med*. 1994;330:592-596.
8. Connors AF Jr, Dawson NV, Desbiens NA, et. al. A controlled trial to improve care for seriously ill hospitalized patients: the study to understand prognoses and preferences for outcomes and risks of treatments. *JAMA*. 1995;274:1591-1598.
9. Donnelly S, Walsh D, Rybicki L. The symptoms of advanced cancer in 1000 patients. *J Palliat Care*. 1994;10-57.
10. Evans C, McCarthy M. Prognostic uncertainty in terminal care: can the Karnofsky index help? *Lancet*. 1985;1:1204-1206.
11. Foley KM. Pain management and palliative medicine in end-of-life patient care. In: *ABIM End-of-Life Patient Care Project on the Identification and Promotion of Physician Competency*. Philadelphia, Pa: American Board of Internal Medicine; 1996:18-23.
12. Hadlock D. The hospice: intensive care of a different kind. *Semin Oncol*. 1985;12;4:357-367.
13. Higginson I. Palliative care: a review of past changes and future trends. *J Public Health Med*. 1993;15:3-8.
14. Johnston G, Abraham C. The WHO objectives for palliative care: to what extent are we achieving them? *Palliat Med*. 1995;9:123-137.
15. Kane RL, Wales J, Bernstein L, et. al. A randomized controlled trial of hospice care. *Lancet*. 1984;1:890-894.
16. Kerr D, Mother Mary Aikenhead. The Irish Sisters of Charity and Our Lady's Hospice for the Dying. *Am J Hospice Palliat Care*. 1993;3:13-20.
17. Kinzbrunner BM. Hospice: what to do when anti-cancer therapy is no longer appropriate, effective, or desired. *Semin Oncol*. 1994;21:792-798.
18. Lamers WM Jr. Hospice: enhancing the quality of life. *Oncology*. 1990;4:121-126.
19. MacDonald D. Non-admissions: the other side of the hospice story. *Am J Hospice Care*. 1989;6:17-19, 40-42.
20. MacDonald N. Palliative care: the fourth phase of cancer prevention. *Cancer Detect Prev*. 1991;15:253-255.

21. MacDonald N. The interface between oncology and palliative medicine. In: Doyle D, Hanks GW, MacDonald N, eds. *Oxford Textbook of Palliative Medicine*. Oxford: Oxford University Press; 1993:11-17.
22. Miller RJ. Supporting a cancer patient's decision to limit therapy. *Semin Oncol*. 1994;21:787-791.
23. Mor V, Kidder D. Cost savings in hospice: final results of the National Hospice Study. *Health Serv Res*. 1985;20:407-422.
24. Mor V, Masterson-Allen S. A comparison of hospice vs conventional care of the terminally ill cancer patient. *Oncology*. 1990;4:85-91.
25. Reuben DB, Mor V, Hiris J. Clinical symptoms and length of survival in patients with terminal cancer. *Arch Intern Med*. 1988;148:1586-1591.
26. Rhymes J. Hospice care in America. *JAMA*. 1990;264:369-372.
27. Saunders C, Baines M, Dunlop R. *Living with Dying: A Guide to Palliative Care*. 3rd ed. New York: Oxford Medical Publications; 1995.
28. Schonwetter RS. Overview of hospice and palliative care in oncology. *Cancer Control*. 1996;3(3):197-203.
29. Schonwetter RS, Teasdale TA, Storey P, et. al. Estimation of survival time in terminal cancer patients: an impedance to hospice admissions? *Hospice J*. 1990;6:65-79.
30. *Standards of a Hospice Program of Care*. Arlington, Va: National Hospice Organization; 1993.
31. Stoddard S. *The Hospice Movement: A Better Way of Caring for the Dying*. New York:Vintage Books; 1978.
32. Storey P, Knight CF. *UNIPAC One: The Hospice and Palliative Medicine Approach to End-of-Life Care*. American Academy of Hospice and Palliative Medicine. Dubuque, Iowa: Kendall/Hunt Publishing Company; 1998.
33. Wallston KA, Burger C, Smith RA, et. al. Comparing the quality of death for hospice and non-hospice cancer patients. *Med Care*. 1988;26:177-182.
34. Walsh D. Palliative care: management of the patient with advanced cancer. *Semin Oncol*. 1994;21:100-106 (Suppl 7).

MODULE TWO

Role of the Medical Director, Staff Physician, and Attending Physician in Hospice and Palliative Medicine

Hospice Medical Director

Medical Directors serve a number of functions in hospice and palliative care settings. Although some common ground exists, hospice programs and palliative care units often differ in their implementation and practice of the role of Medical Director. The nature of the Medical Director's role depends on the organization's size, the Medical Director's job description, and the emphasis a particular organization places on physician involvement. Many hospice programs and palliative care units employ full-time physicians, some employ part-time physicians, and a few rely on physicians who volunteer their services.

Some of the Hospice Medical Director's functions are defined by the conditions of participation included in the Medicare Hospice Benefit (MHB), some are implicit in the hospice concept of care, and others evolve from general organizational dynamics. A basic understanding of the Health Care Financing Administration (HCFA) requirements for Hospice Medical Directors is necessary because HCFA usually provides most of the financial support for hospice programs.

In addition to program-related responsibilities, Hospice Medical Directors often are involved in shaping the future of hospice and palliative medicine locally, nationally, and internationally.

Interdisciplinary Team Role

In hospice and palliative care settings, the hospice interdisciplinary team (IDT) is the vehicle for providing comprehensive interventions. The individual professional identities of members are superseded by their identity as team members. Because the team is the vehicle of action, the interactional process is vital to its success—members share information directly, work together to develop goals, and share leadership depending on the task at hand. Each team member brings a different discipline's perspective to the team. Honoring the professional perspectives of team members is necessary for effective teamwork and for providing quality care for patients and their family members.

Distinguishing between multi-disciplinary and interdisciplinary teams is important. A multidisciplinary team is the work group most commonly used in health care. Team members are recognized first by their professional identities and secondarily by their team affiliation. Traditionally, the team leader is the highest ranking member, usually the physician. Because the team is not the primary vehicle for action, the interactional process is emphasized less and members often share information through the medical record.

The MHB conditions of participation require physician participation on the IDT. As a team member, the physician should not only sign required documents but also meet regularly with other team members to discuss admissions, deaths, recertifications, and issues important to patients and family members. Physicians also understand that their role is not to preside over the team, but rather to participate as a colleague representing the discipline of medicine.

Certification

Before a patient receives Medicare hospice benefits, HCFA requires certification of a terminal prognosis of six months or less, if the disease runs its normal course. The certification requirement is one of the least understood and most distressing elements of the current MHB. To assist physicians, the National Hospice Organization (NHO) developed a very useful publication, *Medical Guidelines for Determining Prognosis in Selected Non-Cancer Diseases*. Whenever possible, NHO used scientific studies of mortality in non-cancer diseases but the guidelines remain a consensus statement that is not yet entirely evidence-based.

HCFA, in conjunction with its fiscal intermediaries, uses the NHO guidelines as the basis for local medical review policies for selected non-cancer diseases. Due to the lack of proven guidelines, physicians may be reluctant to predict the future course of an illness, and wait to refer patients for hospice care until death is imminent. As a result, patients and family members may receive only limited benefit from hospice services.

Hospice Medical Directors should educate physicians about the flexibility of the MHB benefit, in particular the recertification process. Physicians need to recognize that certification and recertification, although in part dependent on a specific diagnosis, are based more on objective parameters of the patient's decline and evidence of disease progression.

Admission

The patient's first certification period begins with admission to the program. The admitting physician and the Hospice Medical Director must both certify that the patient's life expectancy is six months or less, if the disease progresses as expected. Certification is based on information obtained from the primary (attending) physician, supported by the medical record.

Certification rarely requires a pre-admission visit by the Hospice Medical Director; however, the Medical Director or the team physician plays a vital role in developing and authorizing the patient's care plan. It is important to discuss each physician's responsibilities at the time of admission. The attending physician may continue providing primary care, or may ask the hospice physician to participate as a consultant or to assume primary responsibility for the patient. The latter is generally discouraged because it may result in feelings of abandonment on the part of the patient.

Recertification

The MHB currently consists of two 90-day periods followed by an unlimited number of 60-day periods. Patients can continue receiving hospice care as long as they are certified as terminally ill. Recertification of terminal illness is required before one benefit period ends and a new one begins. The Medical Director, the attending physician, and the interdisciplinary team determine the patient's eligibility for continued certification. The process of recertification is valuable; it requires team members to review critically the effectiveness and appropriateness of their interventions.

Education

The Medical Director should serve as a local expert on hospice and palliative medicine. Certification in hospice and palliative medicine, now available through the American Board of Hospice and Palliative Medicine, gives credibility to expert status in the field.

The Medical Director's role as an educator is multifaceted, and important to the continued existence of hospice and palliative care.

The Medical Director's role as an educator includes educating other physicians, physicians' office staff, team members (including volunteers), patients and family members, healthcare professionals not specializing in palliative care (such as home care agency or nursing facility staff), and the community.

Team Education

As a member of the IDT, the Medical Director is responsible for educating other team members about effective medical interventions for terminally ill patients. The Medical Director often educates team members through "mini" inservices during IDT meetings. Usually, the inservices are disease- or symptom-specific. Because they are short, focused, and immediately applicable to a patient's situation, impromptu inservices can be quite effective, with a high level of retention. However, to ensure full professional staff development, other educational methods should supplement the impromptu approach.

Patient/Family Education

The Medical Director should educate patients and families about the disease process, treatment options, the goals of hospice and palliative care, and other issues as required. The Medical Director can provide education directly while visiting patients as the primary physician or as a palliative care consultant, or (indirectly) through staff education and writing educational materials. Most patient/family education is provided by team members during home visits.

Physician Education

Whenever possible, Hospice Medical Directors should educate attending and referring physicians, medical students, house staff, and students of other healthcare professions about hospice and palliative medicine. At a minimum, education should include effective techniques for managing symptoms. General issues related to hospice and palliative medicine should also be included. Educational methods include serving as a consultant

on specific cases, providing sponsored CME activities, and distributing newsletters.

Community Education

The importance of participating in community education should not be underestimated. Community education enhances awareness of hospice and palliative care services, and is likely to increase access to care for patients and families who may benefit from expert palliative care.

Clinical Duties

Many attending physicians want to continue providing direct care for their patients, which is encouraged by most organizations. However, attending physicians may not have adequate knowledge of palliative medicine techniques to provide effective interventions for certain terminally ill patients. In such cases the Hospice Medical Director must serve as an available resource at all times and should promote the use of palliative medicine consultations, often in the form of home visits. Most visits with hospice patients occur in the home setting, due to the patient's diminished capacity; however, some patients can make office visits. The Medical Director can also serve as a patient's attending physician, either by admitting the patient from his or her own practice, or by accepting transfers of patients from physicians who choose not to practice hospice and palliative medicine.

Support of the Team

Although often overlooked, the role of the Medical Director as a support person for the IDT can be very important. The director can help prevent staff burnout and protect team members from the pitfalls and hazards of the medical system. Support should be provided tactfully to avoid developing a negative "us vs. them" attitude when dealing with outside organizations. Supporting the nursing staff is particularly important as they cope with misunderstandings, delays, and sometimes ignorance, while trying to meet the needs of dying patients and their family members.

Ethics

The Medical Director should be competent to provide medical guidance in ethical issues related to end-of-life care. Due to the controversies surrounding some aspects of end-of-life care and the lack of unanimity in the medical community about biomedical ethics, Hospice Medical Directors are likely to be viewed as experts in the field of ethics. Active involvement with ethics committees is desirable, and helps promote a more rational palliative perspective for end-of-life care.

Utilization Review / Quality Assurance / Performance Improvement

The Hospice Medical Director bears ultimate responsibility for the overall quality of patient care provided by the hospice. The MHB assigns responsibility for Utilization Review (UR) and Quality Assurance (QA) to the Hospice Medical Director. The purpose of UR is to ensure a systematic method for monitoring the appropriateness of hospice services and treatments. Included in utilization reviews are issues such as eligibility for admission and treatment interventions, for example, use of foley catheters, parenteral analgesics, and hospitalizations.

Hospice programs usually receive per diem reimbursement for services. In turn, the hospice program is required to meet all of the patient's medical and other needs related to the terminal illness. By participating in UR, the Medical Director can monitor interventions, note those that are ineffective or unnecessarily expensive and replace them in the future with more appropriate palliative measures that may be not only less expensive but also more appropriate for the patient's situation.

Quality Assurance/Performance Improvement (PI) involves the systematic develop-

ment of objective measures of quality, then measuring performance (outcome measures) against those standards. At its most basic level, QA activities include an analysis of the responses of patients, families, and physicians to satisfaction surveys of the program's pain and symptom management interventions, staff attitudes, timeliness, and a variety of other issues. QA also provides a systematic means for reviewing documentation, medication errors, other treatment errors, patient falls, hospitalizations, and other issues that may indicate deficiencies in quality care. Chart reviews and audits are useful ways of assessing quality.

Utilization Review may be the sole responsibility of the Medical Director. More often it is accomplished at the committee level under the direction of the Medical Director. The same hospice committee often deals with UR and QA/PI activities, due to overlap between the two areas.

Administration

The degree to which a Medical Director is involved in program administration, beyond that already described, varies greatly from program to program. The Hospice Medical Director may be expected to serve as an ex-officio member of the hospice's governing body, serve as chair of medical advisory committees, or serve as a department head who credentials, hires, supervises, and evaluates other physicians. Medical Directors should understand the program's expectations regarding administrative positions to ensure the program can provide the necessary resources to fulfill those obligations.

Involving the Medical Director in administrative responsibilities is potentially valuable for hospice programs. Some hospices include the Medical Director in pre-authorizing inpatient care and in authorizing certain types of interventions. Involving the Medical Director in direct utilization review may positively affect the financial viability of the hospice.

Marketing

In many respects, good hospice programs market themselves. Word of mouth from satisfied families is invaluable. Community education programs also increase awareness of and demand for hospice services, particularly when a program's reputation is sustained by high quality care. There is a growing need for directed marketing activities. Ever-increasing numbers of agencies are offering "hospice-like" product lines that may not reflect the comprehensive services offered by hospice programs. The survival of local hospice programs may depend on a critical appraisal of "who the hospice customer is" and which services are needed.

Involving the Hospice Medical Director in marketing and community education may help increase awareness of the program and distinguish it from home care agencies and nursing facilities, which have traditionally defined their Medical Director's role as less hands-on and less active. Direct marketing to physicians is best done by the Medical Director through informal interactions with other physicians. When community physicians see the Hospice Medical Director, they are reminded of hospice care. Formal marketing strategies include publishing physician newsletters, preparing videotapes, and involving the Medical Director in hospital grand rounds and staff meetings.

Research

Although research involving terminally ill patients poses special problems, for example, short survival times, intrusions during a very private time, and obtaining adequate informed consent, it is a vital component of palliative medicine. As in all areas of medicine, research is needed to measure the effectiveness of interventions so physicians can make evidence-based decisions about treatments. Without published research results, the benefits of hospice and palliative medicine will not be recognized by other medical disciplines. In any case, a Hospice Medical Director can be a valuable resource for research.

Hospice Team Physician

As a hospice program grows, additional physicians are needed to provide effective medical supervision and care. Some programs hire an Associate Medical Director, who assumes responsibility for some of the Medical Director's activities. More often, programs employ team physicians who are responsible for team functions and education, allowing the Medical Director to concentrate on administrative and other duties.

Attending Physician

Most hospice and palliative care organizations encourage attending physicians to provide ongoing primary care for their patients after referral for hospice care. This practice lessens the chance that patients or family members will feel abandoned by their physicians. After certifying the patient as terminally ill with a prognosis of six months or less if the disease runs its normal course, the attending physician is responsible for providing and/or approving the admission orders and the plan of care. The attending physician (or his/her covering physician) should be available for consultation and/or orders while the patient is receiving hospice care. The attending physician also signs the death certificate.

Because many physicians are unfamiliar with hospice and palliative medicine, they may require education and support to discontinue medications that are no longer beneficial and to prescribe interventions that will relieve the patient's suffering more effectively. Often the Medical Director makes specific recommendations for patients. Some programs use standing orders, to allow greater flexibility when team members care for patients.

Objectives

Attitudes/Behaviors

1. Discuss the developing role of physicians in hospice and palliative care.

2. Describe methods for achieving timely referrals of patients to a hospice program.

3. Describe issues that should be considered when determining the appropriateness of a particular therapeutic or diagnostic intervention for a dying patient.

4. Defend the provision of comfort care to dying patients as an active, desirable, and important service.

5. Discuss the skills necessary to communicate about death and dying with terminally ill patients, family members, and caregivers.

6. Discuss the skills necessary to communicate about death, dying, and palliative care with members of the patient's healthcare team who are not associated with hospice and palliative care programs.

7. Identify the physician's role on the interdisciplinary team.

8. Identify personal conflicts and anxieties associated with dying that may affect the physician's ability to care for dying patients.

9. Discuss the role of the Medical Director as it relates to UR, QA, and PI programs.

Knowledge

1. Describe five roles of a Hospice Medical Director.

2. Describe three common roles of an Associate Medical Director and/or a team physician.

3. Describe the purpose of the Medicare Hospice Benefit and the process of certification and recertification.

4. List three educational methods Hospice Medical Directors can use when educating various groups.

5. Discuss the uncertainties of prognosis when managing terminally ill patients.

6. Compare the advantages and disadvantages of various care settings for terminally ill patients.

7. Describe the principles of biomedical ethics, including beneficence, nonmaleficence, autonomy, competence, informed consent, advance directives, and guidelines for medical decision making at the end of life.

8. Discuss specific regional laws that impact decision making near the end of life, including requirements for prescribing opiates.

9. Discuss issues of access to comprehensive end-of-life care and financing care for terminally ill patients in various settings.

10. Describe the manner in which appropriateness of enrollment into the hospice program is determined.

11. Describe the responsibilities of the hospice patient's attending physician.

Skills

1. Demonstrate the ability to interact with physicians in ways that encourage timely referrals of future patients.

2. Demonstrate the ability to work effectively with other members of the interdisciplinary team.

3. Demonstrate the ability to educate physicans, team members, and patient and family members about diseases, diagnostic processes, prognoses, medical management, symptom control, and issues related to hope, meaning, and personal growth.

4. Utilize the interdisciplinary team to manage common psychosocial and spiritual problems experienced by patients or family members.

5. Demonstrate effective communication with patients and families.

6. Demonstrate the ability to balance the patient's personal and cultural values, medical factors, and environmental factors when making medical decisions.

7. Demonstrate the ability to help terminally ill patients retain as much control as possible over all aspects of their lives.

8. Demonstrate the ability to conduct and interpret research related to end-of-life care.

9. Demonstrate the ability to control symptoms that threaten the patient's quality of life.

References

1. *About Hospice Under Medicare*. South Deerfield, Mass: Channing L. Bete Co; 1990. Scriptographic Booklet #37796D-10-92.
2. Buchanan, et al. Medical education in palliative care. *Med J Aust*. 1990;152:27-29.
3. Cancer Research Campaign Working Party in Breast Conservation. Informed consent; ethical, legal, and medical implications for doctors and patients who participate in randomized clinical trials. *BMJ*. 1983;286:117-21.
4. Carey RG: Living until death: a program of service and research for the terminally ill. In: Kubler-Ross E, ed. *Death, the Final Stage of Growth*. New York, NY: Simon & Schuster; 1975: 75-86.
5. *Caring for the Dying: Identification and Promotion of Physician Competency*. Philadelphia, Pa: American Board of Internal Medicine: 1996. Educational Resource Document.
6. Charlton R, Ford B. Medical education in palliative care. *Acad Med*. 1995;70(4):258-259.
7. Degner LF, Henteleff PD, Ringer C. The relationship between theory and measurement in evaluations of palliative care services. *J Palliat Care*. 1987;3:8-13.
8. Emanuel EJ, Emanuel LL. The economics of dying: the illusions of cost savings at the end of life. *N Engl J Med*. 1994; 330(8):540-544.
9. Frederich M. Role of the Hospice Medical Director and the Hospice Physician. *Hospice Update*. 1995;5(1):2-7.
10. Greer DS, Mor V. An overview of national hospice study findings. *J Chron Dis*. 1986;39:5-7
11. Kidder D. The effects of hospice coverage on Medicare expenditures. *Health Serv Res*. 1992; 27:195-202.

12. Knight CF, Knight PF, Gellula MH, Holman GH. Training our future physicians: A hospice rotation for medical students. *Am J Hospice Palliat Care*. 1992; 9(1):23-28.

13. Latimer E. Auditing the hospital care of dying patients. *J Palliat Care*. 1991;7:12-17.

14. Martin RW, Wylie N. Teaching third-year medical students how to care for terminally ill patients. *Acad Med*. 1989; 64(7):413-14.

15. McCarthy M, Higginson I. Clinical audit by a palliative care team. *Palliat Med*. 1991; 5:213-21.

16. *Medicare Hospice Benefits: A Special Way of Caring for the Terminally Ill*. Baltimore, Md: Health Care Financing Administration. US Dept of Health and Human Services; 1995. Brochure #HCFA 02154.

17. *Medicare Hospice Manual*. Baltimore, Md: Health Care Financing Administration. US Dept of Health and Human Services; 1985.

18. Olsen SL. Hospice administration, a life cycle model. *Am J Hospice Care*. 1988; 5(1):40-47.

19. Sankar A, Becker SL. The home as a site for teaching gerontology and chronic illness. *J Med Educ*. 1985; 60:308-13.

20. Schonwetter RS, Robinson, BE. Educational objectives for medical training in the care of the terminally ill. *Acad Med*. 1994;69(8):688-690.

21. Scott F, Lynch J. Bedside assessment of competency in palliative care. *J Palliat Care*. 1994;10(3): 101-5.

22. Smith SA, Bohnet N. Organization and administration of hospice care. *J Nurs Adm*. 1983; 13(11):10-16.

23. Stuart B, Herbst L, Kinzbrunner B, Predor M, Connor, S, Ryndes T. *Medical Guidelines for Determining Prognosis in Selected Non-Cancer Diseases*. 2nd ed. Arlington, Va: National Hospice Organization; 1996:1-58.

24. Von Roenn JH, Neely KJ, Curry RH, Weitzman SH. A curriculum in palliative care for internal medicine housestaff; a pilot project. *J Cancer Educ*. 1988;3:259-63.

MODULE THREE

Communication Skills in Hospice and Palliative Medicine

Communication

Effective communication is the first step to successful hospice and palliative care. It helps ensure accurate assessment of a patient's symptoms, better symptom control, and improved understanding of the illness' impact on all aspects of the patient's life, including the patient's family members. Clear compassionate communication is essential to establish therapeutic doctor-patient relationships. Physicians who communicate effectively and compassionately are more likely to develop therapeutic relationships and to understand and address the needs of the entire family system.

Despite the importance of effective communication and the fact that most physicians conduct approximately 120,000 interviews during their careers, physicians receive minimal training in communication. Physicians generally interrupt patients within the first few seconds of an interview and typically spend less than two minutes of a 20-minute session obtaining information. Good communication embodies three general components: accuracy, precision, and effectiveness. Physicians should monitor their communication to ensure they are communicating as accurately, precisely, and effectively as possible.

Effective communication is a process of conveying information and ensuring the receiver understands the intended message.

Because stress and anxiety interfere with the ability to hear and process information, information may need to be repeated several times, particularly when patients, family members, or physicians are upset. Physicians need to remind themselves that the patient's agenda is of utmost importance; until patients are heard, they are unable to listen.

When talking with terminally ill patients about the dying process, common barriers to effective communication include widespread social and personal denial of death, the patient's fears about dying, and the physician's own anxieties about discussing death. In addition, many families lack experience with death and may have unrealistic expectations about the healthcare system's ability to restore a patient's health in the face of a terminal diagnosis. Western society is accustomed to hearing about medical miracles and is less realistic about death than most other cultures.

Practitioners of hospice and palliative medicine should exhibit the following characteristics: attentive listening; commitment to alleviating the patient's pain and other symptoms; interest in exploring areas of personal discomfort when dealing with death, dying, and suffering; acceptance of the inability to always anticipate what will happen next; interest in the meaning of what the dying patient is trying to communicate; interest in the patient's and family's suffering within the context of their individual life experiences; and interest in helping the patient and family explore issues of meaning, worth, value, and hope in the context of a terminal illness.

Understanding the physical, spiritual, and psychosocial dimensions of the dying process is necessary for preparing patients and families for the patient's death. The physical dimension includes a decline in body system functions. When asked, most patients indicate they are much more afraid of what happens during the dying process than of being dead.

Spiritual and psychosocial dimensions include resolving unfinished personal and legal business, resolving family conflicts as much as possible, reconciling estranged relationships as much as possible, searching for meaning (indicated by questions such as, Why me? Why do people suffer? Has my life had any meaning?), and receiving permission from family members to die. Patients and family members also need reassurance that their concerns will be heard and addressed, the patient's symptoms will be treated effectively, and they will not be abandoned.

Strategies for Effective Communication

Two principles are particularly important when communicating with patients and families: (1) the patient is the primary concern, and (2) the family's feelings deserve respectful consideration even when their wishes or instructions cannot be followed. Although the patient experiences the disease, all involved parties experience the illness. Physicians should help patients and family members understand the illness and develop useful responses to it. In some cases, patients resolve their anger and become reconciled to death while family members are still angry and denying the implications of the patient's illness.

In hospice and palliative care settings, communication is important from the moment

the physician meets the patient to the last moment of the patient's life. In the context of hospice and palliative medicine, conversations with patients include two major elements: transmitting medical information and clarifying a patient's feelings and emotions as he/ she responds to the medical information.

Strategies for effective communication in hospice and palliative care settings are simple and practical. They include the following: active listening; using effective nonverbal communication; recognizing the meaning of a patient's and family's nonverbal communication; sharing bad news clearly and compassionately; describing the dying process clearly; communicating openly and honestly with patients and family members; understanding family dynamics; and, most importantly, establishing therapeutic doctor-patient relationships.

Sharing Bad News

Conversations about death and dying can be rather difficult, particularly when physicians must convey bad news about diagnosis or prognosis. In general, physicians are trained to view disease as separate from the person who is experiencing the disease. As a result, they may believe they have little to offer when medical treatments cannot offer cure. Instead, physicans should express feelings of compassion and empathy, which in many situations are more likely to be therapeutic than ordering additional tests or procedures with minimal potential benefit.

When disclosing bad news, key factors to remember include the following:

- Arrange a private meeting place, rearrange furniture if necessary to facilitate communication, and limit distractions as much as possible.
- Introduce yourself to everyone in the room and describe your purpose. Because not all

patients desire physical contact, assess their wishes. When physical contact is appropriate, shake hands with the patient first, then with everyone else in the room.

- Sit down as close to the patient as is comfortable. Sitting down indicates the physician is willing to listen and share control of the situation with the patient and family. Sometimes, sitting just below the patient's eye level diffuses tension when patients are angry or feeling a loss of control.
- If the patient is alone, ask if a friend, family member, or nurse is wanted during the discussion to help the patient remember key points and provide emotional support.
- Assess how much the patient knows, how much he/she wants to know, and whether the news should be discussed now or at a later time.
- Provide information in small doses and in terms commensurate with the patient's ability to understand.
- Ask the patient to share his/her understanding of what has been said.
- When discrepancies exist between what the physician has said and what the patient understands, explore reasons for the misunderstanding.
- Refrain from interrupting the patient and family members. Use gestures, such as nodding and smiling, to encourage the patient and family members to share their understanding of the news and their feelings about it. Allow pauses and learn to be comfortable with silence so they have time to assimilate the news and think of questions to ask.
- Respond to the patient's feelings with empathy, and respect the patient's need to deny the news or close the interview.
- Always follow through. Discuss the next phase of treatment, discuss long- and short-term goals, explain what is likely to happen next, and schedule the next meeting. Reassure the patient of your continued availability.

Family Dynamics

Cancer and other terminal illnesses affect the patient and the patient's entire family system. The patient's experiences are likely to be difficult physically, emotionally, socially, and spiritually, but in some instances the family's experiences may be even more complex. Family members may be able to accept changes in the patient's condition intellectually but they may have tremendous difficulty accepting the illness' implications on an emotional level.

Usually, family members want the following: to be near the dying person; to be helpful to the dying person; to receive assurances about the dying person's comfort; to be informed about the dying person's condition and the imminence of death; to be able to vent emotions in a safe environment; to receive comfort and support from other family members; and to receive acceptance, support, and comfort from healthcare professionals.

Frequently, family systems are described as *functional* or *dysfunctional*. Functional family systems tend to encourage individual freedom of expression and allow freedom to grow and change. They are characterized by the following: clear, direct communication; respect for compromise, mediation, and accommodation; respect for boundaries; receptivity to the ideas of others but selectivity when incorporating new ideas; an ability to work as a cohesive unit; prior successful experience in handling stress; a large and flexible repertoire of coping skills; receptivity to available outside support; and a willingness to perceive difficult situations as opportunities for personal growth and awareness.

Dysfunctional family systems tend to unnecessarily limit and control the actions and emotions of individual members, and are often characterized by strong dependency needs, hostility, or ambivalence. Regardless of a family system's degree of functionality, the family is likely to experience increased stress when one member of the system becomes terminally ill. Family members are likely to experience the following: emotional strain, uncertainty about the patient's care needs, feelings of inadequacy about their inability to provide care, uncertainty about how to comfort the patient, uncertainty about how to respond to the patient's depression and anger, uncertainty about the course of the disease, fear of the dying process, existential concerns, altered roles and lifestyles, altered sexual behavior, changes in finances, and anger about perceived inadequacies of the services provided by outside agencies.

It is important to ascertain how families have dealt with difficult problems in the past. Was one family member the "fixer" of problems? Was the problem openly discussed and dealt with directly? Or, was the problem ignored?

Physician Communication

Even in the best of times, communication among physicians can be rushed, disorganized, and opinionated. However, effective communication is vital and can improve the patient's situation. When communicating with other medical professionals, physicians should emphasize the most important aspects of the patient's situation. For example, before communicating with other healthcare professionals, physicians should ask themselves the following questions: Am I addressing the right person? What do I need to tell the other person to improve the patient's situation? How is the information likely to affect the listener? Who is the responsible party now? Who is going to do what? If problems arise, how do we make contact again?

Stress Management

In hospice and palliative care settings, stress affects not only patients and their families but also the healthcare professionals who care for them. When nurses begin working on palliative care units, their distress scores may equal those of newly widowed women, and may be higher than women undergoing radiation treatment for newly diagnosed breast cancer. As a group, physicians generally are under considerable stress; they have higher rates of first admission for alcohol dependence than controls from a comparable social class, and higher death rates from stress-related causes, such as suicide, cirrhosis of the liver, and drug abuse. Physicians also experience early death from myocardial infarction.

Effective stress management techniques are likely to help physicians better cope with the inevitable stresses that accompany hospice and palliative medicine, and to improve their general sense of well-being. When physicans learn to care for themselves and manage their stress more effectively, they are more likely to provide comfort for patients, seek needed information, discuss their fears and worries, and address problems effectively. Growing evidence indicates that successful coping skills result in less physical discomfort and fewer dependent behaviors such as alcohol abuse. Participation on an interdisciplinary team can greatly reduce the stress of caring for patients and family members, and can provide opportunities for collaboration and support.

Effective stress reduction techniques include the following: muscle relaxation, strenuous exercise, laughter, meditation, prayer, journaling, involvement in meaningful relationships, developing strong spiritual beliefs, recalling positive moments, developing interests outside of work, and participating in activities and situations in which personal individuality is accepted and respected.

Objectives

Attitudes/Behaviors

1. Describe the importance of listening when communicating with patients and family members.

2. Discuss the importance of open and honest communication in therapeutic relationships.

3. Discuss the importance of verbal and nonverbal forms of communication.

4. Describe the likely meaning of common forms of nonverbal communication, including facial and body gestures, postures, and tone or pace of speech.

5. Describe the value of family conferences when conveying information to family members, identifying vulnerable family members, and resolving family conflicts.

6. Explain why a "conspiracy of silence" about a patient's terminal illness may have devastating effects on the entire family system.

7. Explain intellectual versus emotional acceptance of changes in a patient's condition.

8. Describe the importance of family dynamics when dealing with end-of-life issues.

9. Discuss how a physician's own emotional responses to a patient or family may interfere with effective or therapeutic communication.

Knowledge

1. List three objectives when communicating with patients and families about a terminal illness.

2. Describe the range of possible reactions exhibited by patients and families when hearing bad news.

3. Outline strategies for maximizing effective physician-patient communication.

4. Describe strategies for ensuring that the physical setting enhances communication with patients and family members.

5. Describe the goals of effective physician-patient communication.

6. List skills essential to effective communication.

7. Describe specific strategies for improving communication when sharing bad news with patients and families.

8. List stress management techniques that physicians can use to reduce personal stress when caring for terminally ill patients and their family members.

Skills

1. Demonstrate effective and empathic communication skills, including attending, attentive listening, paraphrasing, reflecting feelings, integrating and summarizing, self-disclosure, acceptance, use of silence, and support and reassurance.

2. Convene and facilitate a family interview for the following purposes: data collection, support and reassurance, family education about the patient's illness and prognosis, and family decision making.

3. Use techniques for communicating effectively with patients and families and modify the techniques based on the patient's personal, educational, cultural, emotional, and spiritual background.

4. Demonstrate respect for a patient's or family member's primary values, even when they differ from the physician's personal or professional beliefs.

5. Demonstrate the ability to identify and achieve a specific objective during an encounter with a patient or family.

6. Utilize interdisciplinary collaboration and support when making decisions about patient care.

7. Demonstrate support and reassurance for patients and family members who are feeling abandoned and lonely when dealing with an advanced chronic illness, and provide practical suggestions for alleviating such feelings.

8. Respond appropriately to a wide range of patient/family reactions to news of a potentially fatal illness, e.g., anger, questioning, withdrawal, and blame.

9. Develop techniques for identifying and working with dysfunctional families as effectively as possible.

10. Use effective techniques for communicating distressing information to patient/ families.

11. Demonstrate respect for family structure, beliefs, and values when sharing information and determining treatment goals.

12. Demonstrate an ability to help patients and family members explore spiritual and existential concerns.

References

1. Becker E. *The Denial of Death*. New York: Free Press; 1973.
2. Billings JA. Sharing Bad News. *Outpatient Management of Advanced Cancer. Symptom Control, Support, and Hospice In-the-Home*. Philadelphia: LB Lippincott; 1985: 236-259.
3. Blaer N. Time to let the patient speak. *BMJ*. 1989;298:39.
4. Blanchard CG, Labreque MS, Ruckdeschel J, Blanchard EB. Physician behaviors, patient perceptions and patient characteristics as predictors of satisfaction of hospitalized adult cancer patients. *Cancer*. 1990; 65:186-192.
5. Buchholz W. *Hope, (generic)* JAMA. 1990;263:2357-2358.
6. Buckman R. Breaking bad news: why is it still so difficult? *BMJ*. 1984;288:1597-9.

7. Buckman R. Communication in palliative care: a practical guide. In: Doyle D, Hanks GWC, McDonald N, eds. *Oxford Textbook of Palliative Medicine*. 2nd edition. New York: Oxford University Press; 1996:47-61.

8. Buckman R. *How to Break Bad News: A Guide for Health Care Professionals*. London: Macmillan Medical, 1993.

9. Carr A. In: Hall J, ed. *Psychology for Health Professionals*. London: Macmillan; 1982.

10. Faulkner A, Maguire P. *Talking to Cancer Patients and Their Relatives*. New York: Oxford University Press; 1994.

11. Hall ET. *The Silent Language*. New York: Doubleday; 1959. (Reprinted Anchor, 1981)

12. Hampe SO. Needs of the grieving spouse in a hospital setting. *Nurs Res.* 1975;24:113-19.

13. Hinds C. The needs of families who care for patients with cancer at home: are we meeting them? *J Adv Nurs.* 1985;10:575-81.

14. Holland LC, ed. Now we tell: but how well? *J Clin Oncol.* 1989,7:557-559.

15. Kay P. *Notes in Symptom Control in Hospice and Palliative Care*. Essex, Connecticut: Hospice Education Institution; 1989.

16. Kristyanson LS. Quality of terminal care: salient indicators identified by families. *J Palliat Care.* 1989;5:21-28.

17. Kritsberg W. *The Adult Children of Alcoholics*. Deerfield Beach, FL: Health Communications; 1985.

18. Levitt JM. The conceptualization and assessment of family dynamics in terminal care. *Hospice J.* 1986;2:1-19.

19. Lewis FM. The impact of cancer on the family: a critical analysis of the research literature. *Patient Education Counseling*. 1986;209-89.

20. Maguire P, Faulkner A. How to do it: Communication with cancer patients: 1. Handling bad news and difficult questions. *BMJ.* 1988;297:907-9.

21. Maguire P, Faulkner A. Communicate with cancer patients: 2. Handling uncertainty collusion and denial. *BMJ.* 1988;297:972-4.

22. Maynard D. Breaking bad news in clinical setting. In: Dervin B, ed. *Progress in Communication Sciences*. Norwood, NJ: Ablex Publishing Co; 1989:161-3.

23. McCubbin HI, Patterson IM. Family transition: adaption to stress and the family. In: McCubbin HI, Figley CR., eds. *Stress and the Family, Vol. 1. Coping with Normative Transitions*. New York: Bruner/Mazel; 1983:5-25.

24. Meyerowitz BE, Heinrich RL, Schag C. Helping patients cope with cancer. *Oncology.* 1989;7:557-559.

25. Older L. Teaching touch at medical school. *JAMA.* 1984;252:931-3.

26. Permi J. Communicating bad news to patients. *Can Fam Physician.* 1981;27:837-41.

27. Seravalli EP. The dying patient, the physician, and the fear of death. *New Engl J Med.* 1988;319:1728-30.

28. Sims S. Slow stroke back massage for cancer patients. Occasional Paper. *Nurs Times.* 1986;82:47-50.

29. Storey P, Knight CF. *UNIPAC Five: Caring for the Terminally Ill: Communication and the Physician's Role on the Interdisciplinary Team*. American Academy of Hospice and Palliative Medicine. Dubuque, Iowa: Kendall/Hunt Publishing Company; 1997.

30. Waitzkin H, Stoeckle LD. The communication of information about illness. *Adv Psychosom Med.* 1987;8:180-215.

31. Winslow R. Sometimes talk is the best medicine. For physicians, communications may avert suits. *Wall Street Journal*. Thursday, October 5, 1989 p. B1.

Pathophysiology of Pain

Pathophysiology of Pain

Pain management is one of the most important aspects of palliative medicine. Because different physiological mechanisms of pain frequently coexist in patients with advanced cancer or other chronic medical illnesses, understanding the diagnostic and therapeutic implications of each mechanism is an essential component of palliative medicine.

Further research will identify specific pharmacologic and non-pharmacologic techniques for controlling pain at specific sites. For now, it is imperative that palliative medicine specialists understand the basic components of the neurophysiology of pain, including transduction, transmission, perception, and modulation.

Definition and Types of Pain

The International Association for the Study of Pain defines pain as "an unpleasant sensory and emotional experience associated with actual or potential tissue damage, or described in terms of such damage." The definition acknowledges that pain is physiologically triggered but is mediated by a patient's perceptions and past experiences. Thus, pain is a subjective and unique symptom in every patient.

Traditionally, pain has been classified by characteristics such as severity, pathophysiology, or duration, that is, acute and chronic. The following broad physiological categories of pain are commonly used: somatic, visceral, and neuropathic.

Somatic pain occurs when nociceptors in cutaneous and deep musculoskeletal tissues are activated. Typically, it is well localized and perceived either superficially or in deeper musculoskeletal structures. Somatic pain can occur in patients with bone metastases, post-surgical incisions, and musculoskeletal inflammation or spasm.

Visceral pain results from infiltration or distension of thoracic and abdominal viscera and may occur in patients with liver metastases and pancreatic cancer. Typically, it is poorly localized, described as deep or squeezing, and may be associated with nausea, vomiting, or diaphoresis.

Neuropathic pain results from injury to the peripheral and/or central nervous systems. Pain associated with neural injury often is severe and differs in quality from somatic or visceral pain. It may be described as constant or intermittent. Patients may describe it in terms of burning and/or electric shock-like sensations.

Advances in research have led to improved understanding of the systems involved in the perception, transmission, and encoding of pain. Instead of consisting of rigid structures, pain-related systems are characterized by a plasticity that occurs at various levels of organization, from changes in gene regulation and transcription to changes in structure, function, and connectivity. *Sensitization* refers to the anatomical and pharmacologic changes that take place within the central and peripheral nervous system in response to pain. When sensitization occurs, patients may perceive pain at a lower threshold, pain may occur spontaneously, and the size of receptive fields may change.

Unusual Pain Experiences

The clinical correlates of the nervous system's plasticity may produce unusual pain experiences. *Allodynia* refers to pain resulting from an innocuous stimulus and may be described as mechanical allodynia or warm or cool allodynia. *Hyperpathia* refers to abnormal pain evoked in an area with an increased threshold for sensory detection—the pain is of explosive onset and exaggerated severity, and is characterized by a delay of several seconds. *Hyperalgesia* refers to noxious stimulation perceived with abnormal severity; it is characterized by a decrease in pain threshold, increased pain to suprathreshold stimuli, and pain that is often ongoing. When hyperalgesia exists at the site of a tissue injury, it is referred to as primary hyperalgesia and results from inflammation. When hyperalgesia exists in the surrounding area, it is referred to as secondary hyperalgesia, and involves changes in spinal cord neurons.

Transduction

Transduction is the first step in the pain pathway. Transduction refers to the process by which external noxious stimuli produce electrical activity in the endings of primary afferent fibers. Nociceptors are specific receptors located in skin, muscle joints, and viscera that, when stimulated by injury, convey pain information to the central nervous system. Cutaneous nociceptors are defined morphologically by their appearance in light or electron microscopy. Physiologically, they are defined by their pattern of response to mechanical, thermal, and chemical cutaneous stimuli.

Normally, nociceptors are silent or "sleeping." When a noxious stimulus or injury awakens the receptors, they produce a signal transduction and response. Signals are transmitted by small diameter myelinated A-delta fibers and by unmyelinated C-fibers. Stimulation of A-delta fibers produces a sharp, stabbing pain, while stimulation of C-fibers produces a dull, burning pain. Stimulation of muscle nociceptors typically produces a dull, aching pain. Low-intensity stimulation of visceral nociceptors causes a vague sensation of fullness and nausea, while higher-intensity visceral stimulation produces diffuse pain. Nociceptive fibers terminate in different patterns in various regions of spinal gray matter.

A complex, dynamic relationship exists between the release of chemicals from nociceptive fibers and the release of chemicals from damaged tissues. Chemicals released from nociceptive fibers include Substance P, neurokinin A, calcitonin-gene related peptide (C-GRP) somatostatin, enkephalin, dynorphin, and vasoactive intestinal polypeptide (VIP). Chemicals released from damaged tissues include histamine, serotonin, bradykinin, prostaglandins, thromboxanes, and leukotrienes.

Tissue damage results in a number of events that produce neurogenic inflammation through chemical mediators (e.g., bradykinin and prostaglandins). The mediators can sensitize and activate the peripheral endings of nociceptors. The activation of nociceptors then leads to the release of Substance P, which acts on mast cells in the vicinity of sensory endings and evokes degranulation and the release of histamine. This response directly excites nociceptors. Substance P also produces dilation of peripheral blood vessels. The resultant edema causes a further liberation of bradykinin. Potassium, serotonin, bradykinin, and histamine activate primary afferent fibers.

Normally, several types of pharmacological receptors are located on surface membranes, including opiate, gamma aminobutyric acid (GABA), bradykinin, histamine, serotonin, and capsaicin receptors. With injury, several changes occur in the surface membrane receptors of nociceptor axons, including changes in the effectiveness of specific receptors. For example, under normal conditions, opiate receptors are ineffective in the usual activity of joint receptors; however, they become effective after inflammation develops. Other changes following injury include: (1) production of newly formed adrenoreceptors; (2) up regulation of several neuropeptides, such as VIP and galanin in the dorsal root ganglion and their central branches, but down regulation of other neuropeptides, such as somatostatin, Substance P, and C-GRP; and (3) increased production of neurotrophins and their receptors, which can result in aberrant regeneration and abnormal pain phenomena.

Release of the biochemical substances mentioned above leads to the generation of action potentials and electrical changes in the neuron, thereby effecting transduction of the initial signal.

The clinical implications of the transduction process include interventions that halt or slow the release of chemical cascades. Such interventions alter transduction of the pain signal and reduce or alleviate pain. Various pharmacologic interventions work at this level. Prostaglandin inhibitors such as steroids and non-steroidal anti-inflammatory drugs prevent the release of prostaglandins. Membrane stabilizers such as anticonvulsants and anesthetics inhibit induction of the action potential, preventing further transduction. Capsaicin initially increases the release of Substance P, then depletes it, preventing further transduction.

Peripheral opioid receptor subtypes such as mu (morphine-preferring), lambda (enkepalin-preferring) and kappa (dynorphin-preferring) appear to be located on primary afferents, especially on C-fiber afferents. The autonociceptive effects of opioids can be demonstrated by topically administering an opioid to peripheral tissues at sites of inflammation—the opioid reduces the excitability of the afferent fiber. Interestingly however, opioids do not bind to peripheral opioid receptors in the absence of neurogenic inflam-

mation. Inflammation may lead to production of additional opioid receptors, which indicates that neurons must be "primed" by chemical mediators before opioids have any effect peripherally.

Transmission

Transmission is the process by which impulses are sent from primary afferent nerves to the spinal cord. Projection neurons in the spinal cord transmit the pain message to the thalamus, where it is then transmitted to the somatosensory cortex. Three major anatomic areas are crucial to the transmission of pain: the dorsal horn of the spinal cord, the spinothalamic tract, and the thalamus.

The **dorsal horn** of the spinal cord is where afferent nociceptive neurons (A- and C-fibers) terminate and send their signals to projection neurons. The signals are transmitted by excitatory aminoacids (e.g., glutamate), which bind to the N-methyl-D-aspartate (NMDA) receptors. Stimulation of the NMDA receptors leads to an intracellular influx of calcium and magnesium, and causes depolarization of spinal cord neurons.

Blocking NMDA receptors with drugs, such as ketamine, dextromethorphan, and MU801, reduces wind-up of C-fiber stimulation, and can prevent or terminate central sensitization once it has begun. *Wind-up* refers to an increased response of spinal dorsal horn neurons that occurs due to repeated C-fiber stimulus.

The **spinothalamic tract** is located in the anterolateral segment of the dorsal horn of the spinal cord and can be divided conceptually into two ascending systems—the neospinothalamic tract and the paleospinothalamic tract. The neospinothalamic tract appears to subserve the sensory and discriminatory aspects of pain perception (location and intensity), and the paleospinothalamic tract appears to subserve the arousal, emotional, and affective/suffering components of pain.

Essentially, various components of the spinothalamic tract transmit pain messages to the thalamus and midbrain, along with sensations of cold, warmth, and touch. Some tracts carry signals from the A-delta fibers, which rapidly conduct localized pain and may be important in mediating acute short-lived pain. Other pathways carry signals from C-fibers, which are related to slow, diffuse, emotionally-tinged chronic pain.

Several non-spinothalamic ascending tracts have been identified, including the spinohypothalamic tract, the spinoreticular tract, the spinopontoamygdala tract, and the dorsal column tract.

The clinical implications of transmission are associated with the modulation of pain signals. Specific opioid receptors—mu, kappa and delta—are located in the spinal cord and central nervous system. Opioids decrease the action potential of neurons by decreasing the influx of calcium, thereby preventing or reducing the release of secondary messengers.

Perception

Perception refers to the process that results in the awareness of pain. Pain pathways can be divided into the medial pain pathway, which processes the affective motivational component of pain, and the lateral pathway, which subserves the discriminative component of pain.

Pain signals are transmitted from the ventroposterolateral and ventroposteromedial nuclei of the thalamus to specific somatosensory regions of the cortex. If a signal is blocked anywhere prior to this point, the patient will not perceive pain. Lesions occurring in the cerebral cortex that are large enough to destroy the somatosensory area may produce little or no pain. Subcortical lesions can lead to painful conditions referred to as centrally maintained pain. This condition can occur with injury to the thalamus or spinal cord.

Specific areas of the thalamus influence the discriminative, affective, and motivational aspects of pain. The patient's perception of pain is individualized in the cerebral cortex, where the motivational and affective aspects of pain are determined. The limbic system appears to subserve the motivational, affective, and autonomic components of pain. Limbic involvement is associated with the common signs of acute pain, for example, increased attention, arousal, anxiety, endocrine changes, and increased heart rate and blood pressure. The somatosensory cortex is involved in the discriminative aspects of pain, localization, and intensity.

When patients experience chronic pain, few of the autonomic responses remain present, and patients may not "look" as though they are in pain. Some information about pain is relayed through the brainstem reticular system, which receives spinoreticular inputs. Connections are then made to the hypothalamic, limbic, and neocortical systems. Catecholaminergic inputs to the hypothalamic-pituitary-adrenal axis exert a modulatory effect. The hippocampal and cortical regions receive noradrenergic input exclusively from the locus ceruleus, which may focus attention on painful stimuli and incorporate information relevant to the stimuli.

The somatosensory cortex, the association cortex, and the limbic system all provide input via the release of various neurotransmitters, including serotonin and norepinephrine. Clinical implications associated with perception include the following: alleviating associated symptoms of anxiety and fear; using antidepressants to block the re-uptake of neurotransmitters; and incorporating biobehavioral approaches to pain management such as distraction, education, biofeedback, and imagery.

Modulation

The body's physiologic response to pain signals is to decrease (i.e., modulate) the perception of pain. Modulation refers to the process of decreasing further transmission of pain signals through interactions between afferent ascending pathways and descending pathways in the brainstem and spinal cord. The cerebral cortex and various limbic structures, including the hypothalamus, are components of descending analgesic pathways. Descending pathways terminate in nociceptive sensory projection neurons in the dorsal horn of the spinal cord. These descending pathways inhibit the activity of nociceptive projection neurons through direct connections, as well as through interneurons in the superficial layers of the dorsal horn. The pathways release endogenous serotonin, noradrenaline, and other chemical mediators to suppress afferent nociceptive impulses, thereby modifying the effects of persistent pain. Endorphin-containing interneurons in the periaquaductal gray region and in the dorsal horn play an active role in pain modulation. Serotonin, endogenous opioids, and alpha-2 adrenergic processes also are involved in pain modulation.

Analgesia at the level of the dorsal horn is mediated through the interaction of primary afferent neurons, local interneurons, and descending neurons in the spinal dorsal horn. Primary afferent neurons terminate on second-order spinothalamic projection neurons. Local interneurons containing enkephalin exert both presynaptic and postsynaptic inhibitory actions at primary afferent synapses. The release of serotonin from descending brainstem neurons activates local opioid interneurons, and also suppresses the activity of spinothalamic tract neurons, thus demonstrating the system's plasticity. Alpha-2 agonists such as clonidine provide pain modulation through direct action on adrenergic receptors in the spinal cord, and produce analgesia when delivered directly into the spinal epidural space. Tricyclic antidepressants (TCAs), such as amitriptyline, block the uptake of serotonin and noradrenaline, augmenting their post-synaptic actions in the descending pain-suppression pathways. Opioids are postulated to work on the descending system by contributing to the release of serotonin and other endogenous substances, which then modulate the activity of ascending spinothalamic pathways. Activation of the descending system has been implicated as a reason for the effectiveness of placebo and acupuncture.

Gate Control Theory of Pain

The Gate Control Theory of Pain proposes that neural mechanisms in the dorsal horns of the spinal cord act as gates that can increase or decrease the flow of nerve impulses from peripheral fibers to the spinal cord cells that project into the brain.

The theory postulates that pain is a function of the balance between various types of information travelling into the spinal cord through different nerve fibers. The effectiveness of systemic opioid analgesics may be due in part to activation of the descending analgesia system at specific sites.

Essentially, the dorsal horn is where the pain fibers of the peripheral nerves plug into the central nervous system. It is a complex structure, composed of multiple nerve cells. When stimulated by large fibers not commonly associated with pain, certain neurons can inhibit the propagation of pain. Sensory input is further modulated at successive synapses throughout its course along the spinal cord to the brainstem, thalamus, cortex, and other areas of the brain.

The gate theory of pain focuses on classes of neurons found in the dorsal horn of the spinal cord, such as nociceptive afferent C-fibers, non-nociceptive A-alpha, and A-beta fibers, projection neurons, and inhibitory interneurons. The inhibitory interneurons act spontaneously and normally inhibit projection neurons, reducing the intensity of pain. An inhibitory interneuron is excited by non-nociceptive afferents and inhibited by the nociceptor neurons. In addition to inhibiting the interneuron, the nociceptive C-fiber also directly excites the projection neuron.

Neuropathic Pain

The term "neuropathic pain" is applied to many pain syndromes whose pathology is related to aberrant somatosensory processes that originate with a lesion in the peripheral or central nervous system. Neuropathic pain is defined as pain caused or initiated by a primary lesion or dysfunction in the nervous system. Neuropathic and nociceptive pain frequently coexist; however, due to differing pain mechanisms, they require different treatment interventions. Generally, neuropathic pain responds less well to opioids than nociceptive pain, and is treated using adjuvant analgesics such as antidepressants and anticonvulsants.

Peripheral neuropathic pain stems from injury to the peripheral nervous system and may be characterized by intermittent stabbing and lancinating pain or constant burning pain. Peripheral neuropathic pain includes polyneuropathies and mononeuropathies. Mononeuropathies may be relieved by specific procedures such as neurolytic blockade or decompression.

Central neuropathic pain stems from injury to the central nervous system. Centrally mediated neuropathic pain can be subdivided into deafferentation pain and sympathetically mediated pain. Deafferentation pain includes several syndromes, such as postherpetic neuralgia, phantom pain, and central pain. Interestingly, patients with deafferentation pain have peripheral nerve damage but the pain is sustained by abnormal processes at the spinal cord or brain level.

The gate control theory helps explain why adjuvant drugs such as TCAs frequently are used to treat pain caused by peripheral nerve injury. The site of action of TCAs is not fully understood, but they may potentiate brainstem inhibition of nociceptive transmission at the level of the dorsal horn. They may also have major effects on the ascending monoaminergic systems that project into the forebrain.

The complexity of neuropathic pain illustrates the importance of understanding the gate control theory and the physiologic mechanisms related to the transduction, transmission, modulation, and perception of pain. Treatments for neuropathic pain include not only opioids but also adjunctive approaches that affect specific pain mechanisms. Patients experiencing neuropathic pain may undergo a trial of opioids; however, if pain remains uncontrolled, full consideration should be given to a number of adjunctive approaches, including TCAs, anticonvulsants, steroids, and even neurolytic procedures such as sympathetic blockades.

For more information on neuropathic pain, see Modules Five and Six.

Objectives

Attitudes/Behaviors

1. Explain the concept of neuroplasticity as it pertains to the development of chronic pain.

2. Defend the idea that opioid receptors are part of the naturally occurring pain modulation system, and have no inherent qualities that would distinguish them from other neurotransmitter receptors.

3. Discuss why patients with chronic pain do not look like they are in acute pain.

4. Describe how the modulation of pain can vary between individuals.

5. Discuss the parallel processing of pain by discriminative localizing vs. affective motivational pathways.

6. Defend the use of tricyclic antidepressants in the treatment of neuropathic pain.

Knowledge

1. Describe the different types of nociceptors.

2. Describe the major ascending pathways that transmit nociceptive information from the dorsal horn of the spinal cord.

3. Summarize the descending pain modulation system.

4. Discuss the role of the primary somatosensory cortex in the perception of pain.

5. Identify important cortical areas involved in the motivational, affective, and discriminative components of the pain experience.

6. Understand basic concepts about the neuropharmacology of pain.

7. Explain the mechanisms of action of opiate analgesics.

8. Explain the role of catecholamines in the modulation of pain, including norepinephrine.

9. Discuss the role of important neuropeptides in the modulation of pain.

10. List important agents that activate or sensitize nociceptors.

11. Discuss the effect of tissue damage on nociceptors.

12. Discuss the gate control theory of pain.

13. Describe the differences between A-delta and C-fibers.

14. Discuss the difference between transduction and transmission of stimuli.

Skills

1. Distinguish somatic, visceral, and neuropathic pain when evaluating patients.

2. Discuss the use of NMDA antagonists in the treatment of pain.

3. Discuss the effect of alpha-2 agonists on pain modulation.

4. Describe the pathophysiologic mechanisms by which opioids successfully modulate pain.

5. Manage a patient's neuropathic pain with reference to its pathophysiology.

References

1. Arendt-Nielsen L, Petersen-Felix S. Wind-up and neuroplasticity: is there a correlation to clinical pain? *Eur J Anaesthesiol*. 1995;10 (suppl):1-7.
2. Bernard JF, Bester H, et al. Involvement of the spino-parabrachioamygdaloid and hypothalamic pathways in the autonomic and affective emotional aspects of pain. *Prog Brain Res*. 1996;107:243-55.
3. Cervero F. Visceral pain: mechanisms of peripheral and central sensitization. *Ann Med*. 1995;27(2):235-9.
4. Cervero F, Laird JM. From acute to chronic pain: mechanisms and hypotheses. *Prog Brain Res*. 1996;110:3-15.
5. Chapman DR. Limbic processes and the affective dimension of pain. *Prog Brain Res*. 1996;110:63-81.
6. Coderre TJ, Katz J, et al. Contribution of central neuroplasticity to pathological pain: review of clinical and experimental evidence. *Pain*. 1993;52(3):259-85.
7. Cross SA. Pathophysiology of pain. *Mayo Clin Proc*. 1994;69(4):375-83.
8. Dickenson AH. Central acute pain mechanisms. *Ann Med*. 1995;27(2):223-7.
9. Dickenson AH. Spinal cord pharmacology of pain. *Br J Anaesth*. 1995;75(2):193-200.
10. Dray A. Neurogenic mechanisms and neuropeptides in chronic pain. *Prog Brain Res*. 1996;110:85-94.
11. Eccles J. How the brain gives the experience of pain. *Int J Tissue React*. 1994;16(1):3-17.
12. Elliott KJ. Taxonomy and mechanisms of neuropathic pain. *Semin Neurol*. 1994;14(3):195-205.
13. Herz A. Peripheral opioid analgesia—facts and mechanism. *Prog Brain Res*. 1996;110:95-104.
14. Jacques A. Physiology of pain. *Br J Nurs*. 1994;3(12):607-10.
15. Janig W. The sympathetic nervous system in pain. *Eur J Anaesthesiol*. 1995;10 (suppl):53-60.
16. Lewis KS, Whipple JK, et al. Effect of analgesic treatment on the physiological consequences of acute pain. *Am J Hosp Pharmacy*. 1994;51(12):1539-54.
17. McMahon SB, Dmitrieva A, et al. Visceral pain. *Br J Anaesth*. 1995;75(2):132-44.
18. Mense S, Hoheisel U, et al. The possible role of Substance P in eliciting and modulating deep somatic pain. *Prog Brain Res*. 1996;110:125-35.
19. Ochoa JL. Pain mechanisms in neuropathy. *Curr Opin Neurol*. 1994;7(5):407-14.
20. Pockett A. Spinal cord synaptic plasticity and chronic pain. *Anesth Analg*. 1995;80(1):173-9.
21. Rosenfeld JP. Interacting brain stem components of opiate-activated, descending, pain-inhibitory systems. *Neurosci Biobehav Rev*. 1994;18(3):403-9.
22. Sandkuhler J. Neurobiology of spinal nociception: new concepts. *Prog Brain Res*. 1996;110:207-24.
23. Sawynok J, Reid A. Interactions of descending serotonergic systems with other neurotransmitters in the modulation of nociception. *Behav Brain Res*. 1996;73(1-2):63-8.
24. Siddall PJ, Cousins JJ. Pain mechanisms and management: an update. *Clin Exp Pharmacol Physiol*. 1995;22(10):679-88.
25. Stamford, JA. Descending control of pain. *Br J Anaesth*. 1995;75(2):217-27.
26. Sugiura, Y. Spinal organization of C-fiber afferents related with nociception or non-nociception. *Prog Brain Res*. 1996;113:320-39.
27. Treede RD. Peripheral acute pain mechanisms. *Ann Med*. 1995;27(2):213-6.
28. Vasko MR. Prostaglandin-induced neuropeptide release from spinal cord. *Prog Brain Res*. 1995;104:367-80.
29. Wiesenfeld-Hallin Z, Xu XJ. Plasticity of messenger function in primary afferents following nerve injury—implications for neuropathic pain. *Prog Brain Res*. 1996;110:113-24.
30. Willis WD, Sluka KA, et al. Cooperative mechanisms of neurotransmitter action in central nervous sensitization. *Prog Brain Res*. 1996;110:151-66.
31. Willis WD, Westlund KN. Neuroanatomy of the pain system and of the pathways that modulate pain. *J Clin Neurophysiol*. 1997;14(1):2-31.

MODULE FIVE

Assessment of Pain

Unrelieved Pain

Unrelieved pain is common, especially among patients with cancer pain. Up to 90 percent of patients with cancer experience pain during some part of their clinical course. Pain secondary to HIV disease also is common. Increasingly, patients with irreversible and progressive diseases other than cancer are being referred for hospice and palliative care. Such patients, who often present with advanced renal, liver, or heart failure, chronic obstructive pulmonary disease, or dementia pose special challenges for pain assessment. In hospice and palliative medicine, thorough pain assessments are viewed as the foundation upon which rests effective pain management. This module reviews the components of a thorough pain assessment.

Definitions of Pain

Pain has been defined as "an unpleasant sensory and emotional experience associated with actual or potential tissue damage, or described in terms of such damage." Because pain is subjective, physicians should view individual patients as the experts on their pain experience. The role of the healthcare team is to thoroughly assess pain and skillfully provide effective treatments to manage pain and alleviate distress.

Pain can be acute, chronic, or a mix of acute pain experienced against a backdrop of chronic pain(s). Acute pain often is accompanied by autonomic nervous system changes resulting in the following: anxiety; elevated blood pressure, heart rate, oxygen consumption, respiratory rate, and muscle tension; decreased gastrointestinal motility; mydriasis; and diaphoresis. Patients with acute pain generally look as if they are experiencing pain, for example, grimacing or crying.

Chronic pain, usually defined as pain which persists beyond one month (three months in some research studies), often fails to induce such changes in autonomic nervous system function, and patients may look as if they are depressed rather than in pain. Patients with chronic pain often feel as if pain has pervaded their whole world. Chronic, unrelieved pain can result in clinical depression, sometimes with vegetative signs, especially in individuals who have been suffering for many months or years, and believe there is no end in sight to their pain.

It is not unusual for patients to suffer from multiple types of pain; for example, a patient with newly diagnosed cancer may experience concomitant pain in addition to pain from neuropathy, severe arthritis, or other painful conditions. Patients with irreversible and progressive conditions also may experience pain from other musculoskeletal sources, infection, or myocardial infarction. Patients with cancer may experience several different types of cancer-related pain. All types and potential sources of pain need to be considered during the course of a pain assessment.

Purposes of Pain Assessment

A thorough pain assessment is vital if clinicians are to arrive at appropriate diagnoses and implement effective management plans. The purpose of the assessment is to define all dimensions of the patient's pain, to initiate therapeutic interventions to mitigate disease effect, to minimize distress, and to improve quality of life. A thorough assessment should (1) explore the patient's concerns, (2) identify the pain syndrome and the patient's level of distress, (3) develop a treatment plan, and (4) develop an ongoing assessment plan that includes an assessment tool which works well with a particular patient.

Clinicians should document assessment information in the patient's record and convey it to other team members. Thorough assessments should be repeated with changes in therapy so the clinical team can make appropriate treatment decisions. Emphasis should be placed on determining the therapeutic efficacy of previous or current interventions.

Concept of Total Pain

The concept of *total pain*, developed by Cicely Saunders, Sylvia Lack, and others, recognizes that the experience of pain goes beyond the physiological sensation of pain. Because pain profoundly affects an individual's quality of life, effective pain assessments consider many aspects of the patient's life experience. Total pain encompasses pain experienced in the physical, psychological, spiritual, and social domains. The four domains of pain are interactive; that is, unrelieved physical pain may affect social interactions, sexual function, and role function in the family and community. Spiritual, emotional, and social pain often exacerbate physical symptoms.

To alleviate effectively the patient's total pain, each component of total pain must be effectively assessed and successfully treated.

In addition to pain and other distressing physical symptoms, other contributors to the physical domain of total pain include alterations in functional capacity, strength, endurance, and sleep patterns. The psychological domain of total pain includes feelings of loss of control, somatic preoccupation, memory difficulties, increased anxiety, fear, and depression, and decreased enjoyment and satisfaction. The spiritual domain encompasses hope, religious issues, and concerns about the meaning of suffering and the context or meaning of physical pain.

Pain is inextricably related to the underlying disease process. Previous diagnoses and treatments of underlying disease may have resulted in multiple losses in the patient's life, for example, loss of the sense of autonomy, loss of hope, loss of the ability to perform usual family or community roles, loss of work, and financial losses due to the costs of care. Unrelieved pain exacerbates previous losses and may result in patients' viewing themselves only as financial or emotional burdens to family members.

Because pain is a multidimensional problem that profoundly affects all aspects of a patient's life, physicians should be able to assess the overall situation and define areas needing more focused attention. However, it is unrealistic and inappropriate to expect one healthcare provider to assess adequately and treat effectively all components of total pain. Skilled physicians involve other healthcare professionals with expertise in specific domains of total pain, such as clergy, social workers, and other members of a hospice or palliative care interdisciplinary team, to ensure that patients benefit from a carefully integrated approach to care.

Barriers to Effective Pain Management

Barriers to effective pain management affect healthcare professionals, the lay public, and the healthcare system. Such barriers should be explored carefully and understood, because they often impede effective pain management.

Most practicing physicians and other healthcare professionals have not received adequate training in pain assessment and management. Misconceptions about opioid addiction, tolerance, and respiratory depression are common. Many professionals are uncomfortable using opioids and other pain medications with children or older patients. Several states require triplicate prescriptions, which may lead to underutilization of certain classes of drugs due to a physician's real or imagined concerns about drug enforcement oversight.

Patients and families also suffer from misconceptions about pain and its treatment. Patients often fear the meaning of pain. They may believe increasing or new onset pain signals worsening disease or impending death. Patients may fear that reporting pain will result in further painful diagnostic procedures or interventions such as chemotherapy or surgery. They may believe pain is an expected component of their disease, or fear nothing will be done if they report their pain.

Family members also fear the meaning of pain and are likely to hold their own erroneous beliefs about addiction and tolerance. Because pain is so complex, physicians must view the patient and family as the unit of care and involve other members of the healthcare team in the provision of comprehensive, compassionate interventions.

Some aspects of the healthcare system serve as barriers to effective pain management. For example, in some settings, access to professionals with expertise in pain management may be restricted, effective treatments for pain may be inaccurately perceived as too costly, and the use of appropriate medications to relieve pain may be confounded by social fears of addiction. In addition, the healthcare system does not adequately fund research in pharmacokinetics, pharmacodynamics, and the development of valid, reliable standardized assessment instruments for all domains of pain.

Components of the Pain Assessment

A pain assessment should begin with a thorough history. Patients should be asked to describe each pain in terms of its location, duration, intensity, onset, relieving factors, and impact on lifestyle, mood, and relationships. The assessment should cover all previous complaints of pain, including sites, types, duration of therapy (including nonpharmacologic interventions), outcome of treatment, and limitations on activity.

Special care should be taken when addressing a patient's complaint of allergy to a medication. Patients may have taken one dose of a drug and experienced an adverse side effect such as nausea, about which they were not forewarned and for which the physician failed to prescribe preventive therapy. In such cases, patients may have abruptly stopped the medication because of a presumed drug allergy. Many patients report previous adverse reactions to opioids, often in the postoperative setting. Hypersensitivity and allergies to drugs should be carefully differentiated from untoward side effects, and both should be thoroughly explored to relieve a patient's fears about specific medications.

Because effective pain management cannot occur in isolation from the rest of the patient's medical and psychosocial experiences, obtaining a full medical history is an important part of the assessment process. Past and current diagnoses and medications should be addressed. The family history, social history, and system review provide keys for understanding the patient as a whole person, not just as a disease. Patients (or family members, if the patient is unable to participate) should present all medications the patient is taking, including prescribed and over-the-counter preparations. It is not unusual to discover that patients are taking medications prescribed by multiple providers, who may be unaware of medications prescribed by other physicians. Whenever possible, outdated medications and those no longer medically indicated should be discontinued and discarded, to limit potential adverse drug interactions.

The psychosocial assessment should address the patient's perception of the meaning of pain, psychological symptoms of associated distress, psychological reactions to previous illness, and coping styles and adaptation.

The initial assessment also should include a discussion of the patient's priorities and preferences for treatment options. The patient's wishes may be strongly influenced by past experiences and by religious or cultural beliefs, which may differ from those of the healthcare provider. Pain is not universally recognized by all cultures or religious groups as a symptom to be alleviated or eliminated. Some groups view pain as a rite of passage into the afterlife. For others, pain is viewed as building character and strength of will, particularly among males. Most patients express a desire for full pain relief, but they may or may not be willing to achieve their goal at the expense of loss of mental acuity. Some patients prefer less pain relief in exchange for increased alertness. Such variations in preferences reinforce the need for clinicians to be skilled in therapeutics so all options can be explored, communicated, and subsequently woven into the patient's care plan.

The history should include any past or current problems with substance abuse. Factors associated with this serious problem must be explored. For example, current substance abuse, whether related to alcohol, recreational drugs, or prescribed medications, can interfere with palliative interventions and increase the risk of morbidity and mortality. Clinicians should also explore comorbid physical and psychosocial factors influencing drug use, patterns of abuse behavior, compliance with medical therapies, and the existence of social supports, which may be fragile or nonexistent after years of substance abuse. During the assessment, it is important to determine whether an expert in substance abuse treatment should be included as a member of the patient's care team.

A careful physical examination should be performed with special attention to the neurologic exam, when indicated. The ability to complete a physical evaluation may be limited by the patient's care setting; nevertheless, efforts should be made to perform as complete an initial examination as possible.

During the initial exam, it is important to establish a baseline estimate of the patient's mental status. When changes in mental status occur, secondary to pharmacologic interventions or progression of the underlying disease, they are more readily appreciated if a baseline mental status has been documented. The Folstein Mini-Mental Status Exam often is used for this purpose. The assessment should also explore the patient's psychiatric status. Multiple tools are available for assessing depression, for example, the Yesavage or Hamilton depression scales. However, simple direct questions about the effects of pain on mood may be just as clinically useful. Depressive symptoms may require intervention either before or after pain has been treated.

A pain assessment scale should be used during the assessment to document and monitor pain. Scales commonly employed to document pain intensity include the visual analog scale (VAS), numeric pain intensity scale, and a simple descriptive pain intensity scale. The Memorial Pain Card provides a set of four scales to measure pain intensity using a VAS and a word descriptor scale, as well as a mood and relief scale. The McGill-Melzack Pain Questionnaire is another well known tool for clinical and research purposes; it includes an intensity measure (the present pain index of 0–5), an array of pain descriptors, and a diagram to establish pain location. Many practitioners have developed single-page tools for eliciting information about pain. Simplicity, accuracy, and ease of use must guide decisions about which tool is most appropriate for an individual patient.

When assessing pain pathophysiology, clinicians may need to initiate or review laboratory and radiologic studies to evaluate the clinical problem. If the outcome of a study is likely to affect the patient's plan of care, it should be updated if needed. Sometimes the treatment setting limits the extent of testing.

Identifying the etiology of pain is essential to effective management. Clinicians treating patients with cancer should recognize common types of cancer pain and pain syndromes, including neuropathies, nociceptive pain, bone pain, movement-related pain, and mucositis. Specific syndromes due to peripheral nerve injury include tumor infiltration of a peripheral nerve, post-radical neck dissection, postmastectomy pain, postthoracotomy pain, postnephrectomy pain, post-limb amputation, chemotherapy induced peripheral neuropathy, radiation induced peripheral neuropathy, cranial neuropathies, and postherpetic neuropathies. Because pain syndromes often require specific treatments, they must be correctly identified. For example, patients with peripheral neuropathies, plexopathies, or spinal cord compression may not respond to the typical analgesic ladder approach. Instead, alternative approaches of pain management must be instituted. Prompt diagnosis and treatment of these syndromes can reduce morbidity associated with unrelieved pain.

At the conclusion of the assessment process, discussions should occur between the patient, family, and appropriate care providers regarding the patient's desired treatment goals. Healthcare providers should provide information about techniques and therapeutic options, and facilitate open and honest discussion. Such discussions are helpful not only for clarifying the patient's choices about specific interventions but also for modeling open, honest, compassionate discussion of the patient's condition and wishes. Families are sometimes surprised not only by the patient's concerns and choices, but also by the patient's awareness and understanding of their advanced condition and the desire to discuss such matters. Such discussions can result in productive and healing conversations among patients and family members.

After treatment decisions are made, a plan of care should be developed, discussed with the patient and the family when appropriate, and shared with the entire healthcare team. Follow-up plans should also be included to ensure appropriate ongoing assessment.

Assessing Pain in the Elderly

The majority of hospice and palliative care patients are over 60 years of age. Factors associated with aging can directly affect the accuracy and completeness of pain assessments. Such factors include cognitive impairment, an increased incidence of depression, and sensory limitations that make it difficult to use verbal questioning or standardized tools with small print. In the case of visual or hearing impairment, it is important to ensure that patients can adequately hear the questions posed and clearly see lettering.

Although cognitively impaired elderly patients may slightly underreport pain, their self-reports are no less important than those of cognitively intact patients. An evaluation of five standardized pain assessment tools used by nursing home patients with significant degrees of cognitive impairment (MMSE scores 12.1 +/− 7.9), revealed that print size positively affects a patient's ability to complete the assessment tool. In the study, when large print was used, 83 percent of the patients could complete at least one of the pain scales, and 32 percent could complete all five. The McGill Present Pain Intensity Scale had the highest individual completion rate (65%).

Given the prevalence of medical conditions in the elderly, it is important to list all concomitant medical diagnoses and medications the patient is currently taking, including over-the-counter preparations. Such patients often have experienced previous pain that may have been poorly treated. Previous success or failure of pain management regimens may strongly influence the patient's willingness to discuss pain openly with caregivers. With older patients, as with their younger counterparts, the keys to effective assessment are finding the assessment tools that work best with a particular patient *and* communicating relevant information to all members of the team.

Ongoing Pain Assessment

A complete pain assessment should be performed at admission or during the initial visit, after changes in treatment, and then routinely to monitor the progression of underlying disease and the efficacy of interventions. All team members should use the same assessment instrument with a specific patient. Patients should be encouraged to participate actively in the assessment and monitoring process, with caregiver assistance if necessary. Between assessments by healthcare providers, patients should be encouraged to document their pain using a pain diary, log, or journal to provide additional information, and to assess the effectiveness of the interdisciplinary team's interventions.

At a minimum, patients (or, if a patient is unable to participate, involved family members or significant others) should be asked to

record the date, time, and intensity of each pain, and the effectiveness of pharmacologic or nonpharmacologic interventions. This information allows clinicians to correlate pain reports with medication schedules or changes in interventions. Some pain assessment diaries ask for additional information about pain location, descriptors, changes in bowel pattern, mood, and sleep. Regardless which monitoring tool is used, its format should be flexible enough to maximize information without overtaxing the patient or caregiver.

Pain Assessment as a Model for Assessing Other Symptoms

A complete pain assessment should serve as a model for consistent and continual assessment of all distressing symptoms. For many patients, nausea, vomiting, or dyspnea are equally objectionable or even more objectionable than pain. As with pain, a complete description of each symptom's intensity, location, subjective descriptors, exacerbants, alleviators, and effects on mood, function, and sleep are important factors to be considered.

Objectives

Attitudes/Behaviors

1. Explain the relevance of the concept of total pain.

2. Explain the need for ongoing interdisciplinary team involvement in the assessment of pain.

3. Describe the importance of assessments for both pain and other symptoms in the elderly.

4. Describe the need for adapting assessments to reflect cultural differences and individual patient preferences.

5. Explain the importance of the patient's previous pain history and therapies when completing an assessment.

6. Discuss the importance of understanding different etiologies of pain, as they pertain to the assessment and management of pain.

7. Discuss the effects of unrelieved pain in patients with life-limiting illnesses.

8. Discuss barriers to appropriate pain management, including misconceptions about pain and pain management on the part of physicians, patients, and family members.

9. Explain societal barriers to effective pain management.

10. Defend the importance of exploring a patient's goals and priorities during a pain assessment.

11. Describe several reasons why patients with life-limiting illnesses may underreport or not report pain.

Knowledge

1. Define pain.

2. Describe the purposes of pain assessment.

3. Elucidate the concept of total pain.

4. Differentiate between acute and chronic pain.

5. Describe several barriers to pain assessment.

6. Describe the components of a basic pain assessment.

7. List the basic components of a pain journal or log utilized by patients or caregivers.

8. Describe specific problems that may be encountered when assessing pain in cognitively impaired individuals.

9. Describe different neuropathic pain syndromes commonly experienced by patients with life-limiting illnesses.

10. Describe the components of a physical examination that relate to a pain assessment.

11. Discuss the differences among various pain assessment scales.

Skills

1. Perform a complete pain assessment, including a pain history with special attention to past pain problems, interventions employed, their duration, and outcomes.

2. Explain to a patient or caregiver all of the information that should be recorded in a pain diary.

3. Utilize the pain assessment format as a model for assessing other distressing symptomatology in patients with irreversible and progressive disease.

4. Conduct an appropriate physical examination with special attention to pertinent neurologic exams, mental status, and mood during a pain assessment.

5. Elicit information about pain duration, onset, pattern, and intensity.

6. Determine the etiology of a patient's pain and use it to direct treatment efforts.

7. Elicit a patient's goals and priorities regarding treatment options, and incorporate them in the treatment plan.

8. Utilize special tools and other techniques for pain assessment in the elderly.

9. Communicate with all team members regarding the use of appropriate pain assessment tools for ongoing monitoring.

References

1. Chapman CR, Loeser JD, eds. Issues in pain measurement. *Adv Pain Res Ther*. Volume 12. New York: Raven Press; 1989.
2. Cleeland, CS, et al. Pain and its treatment in outpatients with metastatic cancer. *New Engl J Med*. 1994;330(9):592-6.
3. Cohen-Mansfield J, Marx MS. Pain and depression in the nursing home: corroborating results. *J Gerontol*. 1993. 48(2):96-97.
4. Ferrell BA. Pain management in elderly people. *J Am Geriatr Soc*.1991;39(1):64-73.
5. Ferrell BA, Ferrell BR, Osterweil, D. Pain in the nursing home. *J Am Geriatr Soc*. 1990;38(4):409-414.
6. Ferrell BA, Ferrell BR, Rivera L. Pain in cognitively impaired nursing home patients. *J Pain Symptom Manage*. 1995;10(8):591-598.
7. Foley KM. Pain assessment and cancer pain syndromes. In: Doyle D, Hanks GWC, MacDonald N, eds. *Oxford Textbook of Palliative Medicine*. New York: Oxford University Press; 1993:148-165.
8. Folstein MF, Folstein SE, McHugh, PR. Mini Mental State: a practical method for grading the cognitive state of patients for the clinician. *J Psychiatr Res*. 1975;12:189-198.
9. Hester NO. Integrating pain assessment and management into the care of children with cancer. In: McGuire DB, Yarbro CH, Ferrell, BR, eds. *Cancer Pain Management*. Boston: Jones and Bartlett Publishers; 1995:231-272.
10. Ingham JM, Portenoy RK. The measurement of pain and other symptoms. In: Doyle D, Hank G, MacDonald N, eds. *Oxford Textbook of Palliative Medicine*, 2nd edition. Oxford: Oxford University Press; 1998:203-219.
11. Jacox AK, Carr DB, Payne R, et al. *Management of Cancer Pain*. Clinical Practice Guideline Number 9. Agency for Health Care Policy and Research. US Department of Health and Human Services. Publication No. 94-0592. March 1994:7-38.
12. Jensen MP, Karoly P. Self-report scales and procedures for assessing pain in adults. In: Turk DC, Melzack R, eds. *Handbook of Pain Assessment*. New York: Guilford Press; 1992:135-151.
13. Katz S, Downs TD, Cash HR, Grotz, RC. Progress in development of the Index of ADL. *Gerontologist*. 1970;10(1):20-30.
14. Levy MH. Pharmacologic treatment of cancer pain. *New Engl J Med*. 1996;335(15):1124-1132.
15. McGuire DB. The multiple dimensions of cancer pain: a framework for assessment and management. In: McGuire DB, Yarbro CH, Ferrell BR, eds. *Cancer Pain Management*. Boston: Jones and Bartlett Publishers; 1995:1-17.
16. Melzack R, Katz J. Pain measurement in persons with pain. In: Wall PD, Melzack R, eds. *Textbook of Pain*. New York: Churchill Livingstone; 1994:337-351.
17. Melzack R, Katz, J. The McGill Pain Questionnaire: appraisal and current status. In: Turk DC, Melzack R, eds. *Handbook of Pain Assessment*. New York: Guilford Press; 1992: 152-168.
18. Pain measurement in humans. In: Fields HL, ed. *Core Curriculum for Professional Education in Pain*, 2nd edition. Seattle: International Association for the Study of Pain Press; 1995:9-12.
19. Parmelee PA, Katz IR, Lawton MP. The relation of pain to depression among the institutionalized aged. *J Gerontology*. 1991;46(1):15-21.
20. Parmelee PA, Smith B, Katz IR. Pain complaints and cognitive status among elderly institution residents. *J Am Geriatr Soc*. 1993;41(5):517-522.
21. Passik SD, Portenoy RK. Substance abuse issues in palliative care. In: Berger A, ed. *Principles and Practice of Supportive Oncology*. Philadelphia: Lippincott-Raven Publishers; 1988;513-529.

22. Portenoy RK, Kanner RM. Definition and assessment of pain. In: Portenoy RK, Kanner RM, eds. *Pain Management: Theory and Practice*. Contemporary Neurology Series. Philadelphia: FA Davis Company; 1996:3-18.

23. Price DD, Harkins, SW. Psychophysical approaches to pain measurement and assessment. In: Turk DC, Melzack R, eds. *Handbook of Pain Assessment*. New York: The Guilford Press: 1992:111-134.

24. *Principles of Analgesic Use in the Treatment of Acute Pain and Cancer Pain*. Skokie, Ill: American Pain Society; 1992.

25. Stein, WM. Cancer pain in the elderly. In: Ferrell BR, Ferrell, BA, eds. *Pain in the Elderly*. Seattle: International Association for the Study of Pain Press. 1996:69-80.

26. Stein WM, Ferrell, BA. Pain in the nursing home. *Clinic Geriatric Med*. 1996;12(3):601-613.

27. Stein WM, Miech, RP. Cancer pain in the elderly hospice patient. *J Pain Symptom Manage*. 1993. 8(7):474-482.

28. Storey P, Knight CF. *UNIPAC Three: Assessment and Treatment of Pain in the Terminally Ill*. American Academy of Hospice and Palliative Medicine. Dubuque, Iowa: Kendall/Hunt Publishing Company; 1996:1-15,51-82.

29. Turk DC, Melzack R. The measurement of pain and the assessment of people experiencing pain. In: Turk DC, Melzack R, eds. *Handbook of Pain Assessment*. New York: The Guilford Press: 1992:3-12.

MODULE SIX

Pain Management

Goals of Pain Management

Unrelieved pain is a common cause of suffering. A patient's perception of pain depends on complex interactions between nociceptive and non-nociceptive impulses, underscoring the need for comprehensive approaches to treating pain. The goals of comprehensive pain management include analgesia, relief of suffering, modulation of side effects, and patient involvement with and commitment to an effective analgesic regimen. A successful pain management regimen also prevents loss of cognitive function, enhances independence, and improves the patient's quality of life as much as possible.

No one best approach to effective pain management exists. Instead, pain management plans must be individualized based on the patient's stage of disease, comorbidities, and psychosocial and cultural characteristics. Plans should also include counseling patients about achievable goals, for example, first achieving a pain-free, restful night's sleep, then being pain free at rest, then being pain free with movement.

Successful pain management plans recognize the physiological, psychosocial, spiritual, and social contributors to pain, and include both pharmacologic and non-pharmacologic therapies. For example, physiological changes associated with aging that affect pharmacokinetics in the elderly include changes in body composition (decreases in total body water),

declining organ function (decreasing creatinine clearance), and loss of functional reserve (vital capacity). Psychosocial issues affecting a patient's perception and expression of pain include past experiences with the healthcare system, cultural relationships, ethnicity, and socioeconomic status; for example, the cost of medications and treatments may prevent patients from reporting pain until late in the course of the illness, or from obtaining adequate pain relief at all. After a comprehensive initial evaluation, treatment plans should be reassessed continually, and revised when dictated by changes in the patient's condition.

Treatment of Pain

In cancer patients, 60 to 80 percent of pain results from direct tumor involvement with soft tissue and bone, 20 to 25 percent of pain results from cancer treatments themselves, and 3 to 10 percent of pain is due to unrelated comorbidities. Whenever possible, every effort must be made to eliminate the causes of pain. Even in hospice settings, certain types of surgical procedures, chemotherapy, and radiation therapy treatments may provide substantial relief of pain with minimal treatment-related morbidity. Pharmacologic therapy represents the mainstay of effective pain management, but usually must be combined with non-pharmacologic interventions to truly optimize pain relief.

Pharmacologic Treatment

The World Health Organization's (WHO) three-step analgesic ladder provides a useful guide for treating pain. It also incorporates important principles for effective pharmacologic treatment of pain, including the following: (1) as pain increases, effective analgesia requires switching from nonopioids to weak opioids to strong opioids; (2) adjuvant medications often are necessary to control pain; (3) the oral route should be used whenever possible due to general tolerability, ease of delivery, and cost; (4) medications should be given around the clock for chronic pain, not on an "as needed" basis; (5) additional doses of medication should be available to control breakthrough and incident pain; (6) pharmacologic treatments should be based on the pain's specific etiology, which requires careful assessment to identify the cause(s) of each pain; and (7) perceptions of pain vary tremendously, requiring individualized treatment plans for each patient and for each type of pain.

Non-opioid Analgesics

Non-opioid analgesics such as acetaminophen, aspirin, and other non-steroidal anti-inflammatory drugs (NSAIDs) are the treatments of choice for mild pain. Non-opioid analgesics are the first step on the WHO pain treatment ladder, and provide a base on which other agents may be added as needed.

Aspirin and acetaminophen are the most commonly used non-opioid analgesics. Unlike aspirin and other NSAIDs, acetaminophen does not possess significant anti-inflammatory properties. Because inflammation plays a major role in many pain syndromes, acetaminophen may not be the drug of choice in some cases. NSAIDs function as prostaglandin inhibitors by inhibiting cyclooxygenase. Bone pain due to metastasis is thought to be mediated, in part, by prostaglandins. Practitioners typically prescribe NSAIDs for the treatment of mild pain caused by malignancies.

In addition to aspirin, at least fifteen other NSAIDs from five classes are available in the United States. NSAIDs vary according to half-life, duration of analgesic action, and time to peak of pain relief, but there is no evidence supporting superior safety or analgesia of one agent over another or of aspirin over any other NSAID. NSAIDs demonstrate a "ceiling effect" in their analgesic potential; that is, above a certain dose, further escalation provides no additional efficacy. The initial choice of a NSAID should be based on efficacy, safety, relative expense of the medication, patient preference, and compliance. NSAID dosing should be titrated as needed and tolerated for analgesic efficacy, to the maximum analgesic ceiling.

When one class of NSAID does not provide effective relief, a NSAID from a different class should be tried. When initiating NSAID therapy, a baseline hematocrit, BUN and/or creatinine should be considered. Subjective complaints of gastrointestinal upset should be carefully evaluated. Possible adverse side effects include gastrointestinal problems (gastric ulceration), platelet abnormalities (inhibition of platelet aggregation), hepatic dysfunction, renal toxicity (renal insufficiency or renal failure), and fluid retention.

Weak Opioids

Based on the specific receptors to which they bind and their intrinsic activity at receptor sites, opioids are classified as full agonists, partial agonists, or mixed agonist/antagonists. Because some agonist/antagonist opioids offer minimal analgesic benefit, full agonists are the recommended treatments of choice. (Substituting a mixed agonist/antagonist opioid for a full agonist can cause withdrawal symptoms.) Opioids provide analgesia by binding to specific receptors both inside and outside the central nervous system.

When non-opioid analgesics prove ineffective, adding a weak opioid is the next step in the WHO treatment ladder. Codeine is the most commonly used weak opioid due to its widespread availability and reasonable cost. Propoxyphene is a relatively poor agent and is no more effective than NSAIDs. Many combination formulations are available; typically they combine non-opioids such as acetaminophen or aspirin with opioids such as codeine, hydrocodone, or oxycodone. Dosages of combination products are limited due to the potential toxicity of the non-opioid medication. Although oxycodone has been described as a weak opioid due to dose limitations when it is combined with acetaminophen or aspirin, it has at least the same potency as morphine and can be titrated to high doses as a single agent. Thus, oxycodone can be considered a strong opioid.

Strong Opioids

Strong opioids comprise the third step of the WHO pain ladder. When moderate to severe pain is not controlled with weaker opioids, or when other agents cause intolerable side effects, strong opioids are recommended. When used alone, opioids have no upper ceiling effect; however, high dosages of some agents may be limited by intolerable side effects. Commonly used strong opioids include morphine, oxycodone, hydromorphone, fentanyl, levorphanol, and methadone.

Morphine continues to be the opioid of choice for patients with moderate to severe cancer pain. Because morphine is so commonly used, it is available in many formulations, including sustained-release preparations and concentrated immediate-release solutions. Caution is required when using strong opioids in patients with impaired renal function, as some have active metabolites that can accumulate and lead to toxicity. Such patients should be observed closely.

Oxycodone is an effective opioid for controlling severe pain, and is available in controlled release formulations. Fentanyl is available in transdermal formulations. Preparations of meperidine and pentazocine should not be used due to their side effects and relatively poor bioavailability when given

orally. Normeperidine, a metabolite of meperidine, can accumulate, resulting in central nervous system excitability and seizures. Although relatively inexpensive, methadone is difficult to use due to its extremely long half-life and the metabolites formed during biodegradation.

When using strong or sustained-release opioids, physicians should provide rescue or "as-needed" doses of an immediate-release formulation to control episodes of escalating or breakthrough pain. The immediate-release rescue dose should be approximately 15 percent to 25 percent of the total daily dose of the sustained-release product, and should be given every two to four hours as needed. If more than one rescue dose is required in a twenty-four hour period, appropriate increases should be made in the dosage of the sustained-release preparation.

Concerns About Opioids

When opioid therapy is initiated, nausea and somnolence may be common though transient side effects. Nausea can be controlled with agents such as prochlorperazine or haloperidol, given for the first few days of therapy. Constipation is the most common side effect of opioid treatment, and does not abate with long-term use of opioids. Before initiating opioid therapy, the patient's bowel habits must be carefully assessed. When the patient is already using laxatives, has a known history of drug-induced constipation, or is passing fissured or cracked stools, an effective bowel regimen should be initiated when opioid therapy begins. A bowel stimulant and stool softener should be given in effective doses. Itching may result from a nonspecific histamine response to an opioid. It is usually short-lived and can be managed by an antihistamine or by rotating opioids. Clinically significant respiratory depression is also rare when opioids are titrated appropriately.

Chronic opioid use is associated with physical dependence, which differs from psychological dependence or addiction.

Addiction is manifested by drug abuse and inappropriate drug-seeking behavior. When opioids are stopped abruptly, both addicts and patients using opioids chronically for pain management experience similar physical signs and symptoms of withdrawal, including drenching sweats, abdominal cramps, malaise, and dread. Withdrawal symptoms can be avoided by decreasing the total daily dose of the opioid by 25 percent each day until effective opioid dosing is obtained or the patient no longer requires opioid therapy.

Opioid tolerance is characterized by a gradual decrease in analgesic effect; its cause is unknown. For patients with pain, particularly those with cancer-associated pain, the need for higher dosages of medication to achieve adequate relief of pain is typically associated with disease progression, not pharmacologic tolerance. Opioid tolerance and physical dependence do not indicate addiction. Education about effective and appropriate uses of opioids and the differences between addiction and tolerance is critical not only for lay people but also for healthcare professionals.

Adjuvant Medications

Adjuvant medications can be used during each step of the WHO pain treatment ladder to enhance the analgesic efficacy of opioids, to treat concurrent symptoms that exacerbate pain, and to provide independent analgesia for certain types of pain. Commonly used adjuvant medications include corticosteroids, anticonvulsants, neuroleptic agents, and tricyclic antidepressants.

Corticosteroids are used to elevate mood, stimulate appetite, control nausea and vomiting, reduce inflammation, decrease intracranial pressure, and relieve spinal cord compression. Anticonvulsants are used to control neuropathic pain having a lancinating or electric quality. Tricyclic antidepressants are also useful adjuvants for treating cancer pain, particularly neuropathic pain with a burning quality. Neuroleptic agents also serve as adjuvant analgesics for the management of neuropathic pain. Other medications commonly used as adjuvants include antihistamines, local anesthetics, antiarrythmics, and psychostimulants.

Alternative Delivery Routes

When patients are unable to take medications orally, satisfactory levels of pain control usually can be achieved with alternative, noninvasive routes, for example, sublingual, buccal, vaginal, rectal, and transdermal. The transdermal route of absorption may be impacted by physiological changes associated with a patient's illness, such as fever and diaphoresis. Its application at high doses is limited by body surface area. In addition to opiate suppositories, many oral opioids can be given via the rectal route. When changing patients from the oral to the rectal route, begin with the patient's oral dosage and titrate as needed.

Patient-controlled analgesia (PCA) often is used for pain control in acute care settings, but continuous infusions provide the most consistent level of analgesia for chronic pain. Subcutaneous administration of opioids provides effective pain control and achieves blood levels similar to those obtained with intravenous administration. Intravenous delivery is easily accomplished when patients already have permanent intravenous access for other reasons. Remember the importance of equianalgesic dosing when changing to and from parenteral routes. When pain remains uncontrolled or side effects are intolerable, analgesics can be delivered intraspinally. Frequent intramuscular injections should be avoided; they are rarely necessary and cause undue pain.

Invasive Techniques

Invasive techniques for delivering medication should only be used when a noninvasive route proves ineffective. Less than 5 percent of patients with cancer pain require invasive techniques to relieve pain. In selected patients, surgical procedures may be useful to debulk tumors and reduce symptoms associated with obstruction or compression. Anesthetic (nerve blocks) or neurosurgical methods (neuro-ablation, implantation of drug infusion systems, and neuroaugmentation) can be used to ablate pain pathways and to implant devices for delivering drugs or electrically stimulating neural structures.

Non-pharmacologic Treatments

To achieve optimum pain control, non-pharmacologic interventions can be used concurrently with pharmacologic therapy. Non-pharmacologic interventions may include radiation or physical and psychosocial therapies which in many cases can be pro-vided not only by professional staff but also by friends, family members, and sometimes by patients themselves. Often, patients are motivated to use physical and psychosocial therapies because they enhance the patient's sense of control over the illness and encourage active participation in self-care activities.

Physical modalities encompass treatments such as cutaneous stimulation (including massage therapy), exercise, transcutaneous electrical nerve stimulation (TENS), and acupuncture. Psychosocial modalities include cognitive and/or behavioral techniques, relaxation, imagery, distraction, patient education, psychotherapy (individual or group), and hypnosis. One of the primary goals of psychosocial intervention is to help patients gain a sense of control over their perception of pain. Cognitive techniques can influence a patient's perception of pain, which may alter their sensitivity to pain, change their feelings about the pain, and modify their reactions to pain. Behavioral techniques help patients develop skills to cope with and modify their reactions to pain.

Objectives

Attitudes/Behaviors

1. Describe how psychological, social, economic, cultural, and spiritual factors affect a patient's perception of pain and acceptance of pain management treatment plans.

2. Discuss the effects of uncontrolled pain on the family system.

3. Explain misconceptions about pain and its management, and how they affect pain management treatment plans.

4. Discuss professional attitudes toward pain management and how they affect patient care.

5. Discuss the role of adjuvant medications when managing patients with pain, particularly patients using opioids to control severe pain.

6. Describe the relationship between pain and depression.

7. Defend the effectiveness of the WHO analgesic ladder when treating pain.

8. Explain the importance of subjectivity and attention to detail when evaluating and treating a patient's pain.

9. Explain the effects of pain on the quality of life of terminally ill patients.

10. Explain the importance of equianalgesic dosing.

11. Discuss the limitations of certain pain management therapies in the home setting.

12. Discuss the importance of using pharmacologic and non-pharmacologic methods when managing pain.

13. Describe clinical indications requiring invasive pain management techniques.

Knowledge

1. Describe appropriate drugs and their pharmacology for treating the following pain syndromes: bone pain, nociceptive pain, neuropathic pain, visceral pain, increased intracranial pressure, distention and/or compression, and muscle pain.

2. Describe the use of non-pharmacologic methods when managing the above pain syndromes.

3. Describe the use of disease-altering therapies (hormonal therapies, radiation, etc.) for the particular pain syndromes described above.

4. Explain the risks and benefits of invasive modalities (PCA pumps, epidural and intrathecal catheters) for treating pain in patients with advanced disease.

5. Explain the WHO analgesic ladder approach to the treatment of pain.

6. Describe indications, contraindications, and mechanisms of action for aspirin, NSAIDs, and opioids in the treatment of pain.

7. Describe routes of administration, side effects, cost, and common drug interactions of the above medications when used to control pain.

8. Discuss the management of breakthrough pain and incident pain.

9. Describe several non-pharmacologic approaches for managing pain, including psychosocial and physical modalities.

10. Explain the use of invasive therapies (drug infusions, rhizotomy, etc.) in the treatment of pain.

11. Describe specific groups of adjuvant medications and their indications.

12. Explain the difference between dependence, addiction, and tolerance.

Skills

1. Write complete pain management orders for patients with advanced diseases.

2. Calculate equianalgesic dosing when changing a patient's drug regimen.

3. Collaborate with the interdisciplinary team to optimize pain management from a multidisciplinary perspective.

4. Incorporate the use of adjuvant medications in the treatment of pain.

5. Treat pain in patients from various age groups, e.g., pediatrics to geriatrics.

6. Use appropriate medications/dosages for treatment of breakthrough pain.

7. Use appropriate dosing intervals based on medication regimens and patient compliance.

8. Choose effective medications for managing pain based on efficacy, compliance, and cost.

9. Continuously monitor the effectiveness of treatments for the following pain syndromes: bone pain, nociceptive pain, neuropathic pain, visceral pain, increased intracranial pressure, and muscle pain.

10. Incorporate non-pharmacologic approaches when treating pain.

References

1. Baillie SP, Bateman DN, Coates PE, Woodhouse KW. Age and the pharmacokinetics of morphine. *Age Ageing.* 1989;18:258-62.
2. Barbour LA, McGuire DB, Kirchhoff KT. Nonanalgesic methods of pain control used by cancer outpatients. *Oncol Nurs Forum.* 1986;13:56-60.
3. Bonica JJ, ed. *The Management of Pain.* Philadelphia: Lea & Febiger; 1990.
4. Breitbart W, Passik SD. Psychological and psychiatric interventions in pain control. In: Doyle D, Hanks GWC, MacDonald N, eds. *Oxford Textbook of Palliative Medicine.* New York: Oxford University Press; 1993:244-256.
5. Brescia F, Adler D, Gray G, et al. Hospitalized advanced cancer patients: a profile. *J Pain Symptom Manage.* 1990;5:221-227.
6. Chrischilles EA, Lemke JH, Wallace RB, Drube GA. Prevalence and characteristics of multiple analgesic use in an elderly study group. *J Am Geriatr Soc.* 1990;38:979-984.
7. Devulder J, Ghys L, Dhondt W, Rolly G. Spinal analgesia in terminal care: risk versus benefit. *J Pain Symptom Manage.* 1994;9(2):75-81.
8. Emanuel, EJ. Pain and symptom control: patient rights and physician responsibilities. *Hematol Oncol Clin North Am.* 1996;10:41-57.
9. Ferrell, BA. Pain management in elderly people. *J Am Geriatric Society.* 1991;39:64-73.
10. Ferrell BA, Bradley LA, Cooney LM, et al. The management of chronic pain in older persons. AGS Panel on Chronic Pain in Older Persons. *J Am Geriatric Society.* 1998;46:635-651.
11. Ferrell BR, Ferrell BA. Pain in elderly persons. In: McGuire DB, Yarbro CH, Ferrell B, eds. *Cancer Pain Management.* Boston: Jones & Bartlett; 1995:273-289.
12. Foley KM. Management of cancer pain. In: DeVita VT, Hellman S, Rosenberg SA, eds. *Cancer: Principles and Practice of Oncology.* 4th ed. Philadelphia: Lippincott; 1993:2417-2448.
13. Foley KM. Pain assessment and cancer pain syndromes. In: Doyle D, Hanks GW, MacDonald N, eds. *Oxford Textbook of Palliative Medicine.* New York: Oxford University Press; 1993:148-165.
14. Foley KM. Pain syndromes in patients with cancer. *Med Clin North Am.* 1987;71:169-184.
15. Hanks GWC, Portenoy RK, MacDonald N, O'Neill WM. Difficult pain problems. In: Doyle D, Hanks GW, MacDonald N, eds. *Oxford Textbook of Palliative Medicine.* New York: Oxford University Press; 1993:257-274.
16. Hays H, Hagen N, Thirwell M, Dhaliwal H, et al. Comparative clinical efficacy and safety of immediate release and controlled release hydromorphone for chronic severe cancer pain. *Cancer.* 1994;74:1808-1816.
17. Hill CS, Fields WS. Drug treatment of cancer pain in a drug oriented society. In: *Advances in Pain Research and Therapy,* eds. New York: Raven Press; 1989.
18. Jacox A, Carr DB, Payne R, et al. *Management of Cancer Pain. Clinical Practice Guideline No. 9.* AHCPR Publication N. 94-0592. Rockville, MD. Agency for Health Care Policy and Research, U.S. Department of Health and Human Services, Public Health Service; March 1994:8.

19. Loscalzo M, Jacobsen PO. Practical and behavioral approaches to the effective management of pain and distress. *J Psychosoc Oncol.* 1990;8:139-169.
20. McGuire DB, Yarbro CH, Ferrell BR, eds. *Cancer Pain Management.* Boston, Mass: Jones and Bartlett; 1995.
21. Pace V. Use of nonsteroidal anti-inflammatory drugs in cancer. *Palliat Med.* 1995;9:273-286.
22. Parmelee, PA. Pain in cognitively impaired older persons. *Clin Geriatr Med.* 1996;12:473-489.
23. Portenoy RK. Adjuvant analgesics in pain management. In: Doyle D, Hanks GW, MacDonald N, eds. *Oxford Textbook of Palliative Medicine.* New York: Oxford University Press; 1993:187-203.
24. Portenoy RK. Adjuvant analgesic agents. *Hematol Oncol Clin North Am.* 1996;10:103-121.
25. Portenoy RK. Neuropathic pain. In: Portenoy RD, Kanner RM, eds. *Pain Management: Theory and Practice.* EA Davis: Philadelphia; 1996: 83-125.
26. Portenoy RK, Hagen NR. Breakthrough pain: definition, characteristics and prevalence. *Pain.* 1990;41:273-281.
27. Porter J, Jick H. Boston Collaborative Drug Surveillance Program. Addiction rare in patients treated with narcotics. *N Engl J Med.* 1980;302(2):123. Letter.
28. Raj PP. Local anesthetic blockade. In: Patt RB, ed. *Cancer Pain.* Philadelphia: Lippincott; 1993:329-341.
29. Raskin JB, White RH, Jackson JE, et al. Misoprostol dosage in the prevention of nonsteroidal anti-inflammatory drug induced gastric and duodenal ulcers: a comparison of three regimens. *Ann Intern Med.* 1995;123:344-350.
30. Rhiner M, Ferrell BR, Ferrell BR, et al. A structured non-drug intervention program for cancer pain. *Cancer Prac.* 1993;1:137.
31. Roche RJ, Forman WB. Pain management for the geriatric patient. *Clin Podiatr Med.* 1994;11:10-13.
32. Schofferman J. Long term use of opioid analgesics for the treatment of chronic pain of nonmalignant origin. *J Pain Symptom Manage.* 1993;8:279-288.
33. Storey P. More on the conversion of transdermal fentanyl to morphine. *J Pain Symptom Manage.* 1995;10(8):581.
34. Storey P, Hill HH, St. Louis RH, Tarver EE. Subcutaneous infusions for control of cancer symptoms. *J Pain Symptom Manage.* 1990;5:33-41.
35. Twycross R. Misunderstandings about morphine. In: Twycross R, ed. *Pain Relief in Advanced Cancer.* New York: Churchill Livingston; 1994:333-347.
36. Twycross RG, Lack SA. *Oral Morphine in Advanced Cancer.* 2nd edition. Beaconsfield, Bucks, England: Beaconsfield Pubs., Ltd; 1993.
37. Von Roenn JH, Cleeland CS, Gonin R, et al. Physician attitudes and practice in cancer pain management: a survey from the Eastern Cooperative Oncology Group. *Ann Intern Med.* 1993;119:121-126.
38. Waldman SD, et al. Intraspinal opioid therapy. In: Patt RB, ed. *Cancer Pain.* Philadephia: JB Lippincott; 1993:285-328.
39. Warfield, CA. Guidelines for routine use of controlled release oral morphine sulfate tablets. *Semin Oncol.* 1993;20(1):36-47.
40. Watanabe S, Bruera E. Corticosteroids as adjuvant analgesics. *J Pain Symptom Manage.* 1994;9:442-445.
41. Wilkinson TJ, Robinson BA, Begg EJ, Duffull SB, Ravenscroft PJ, Schneider JJ. Pharmacokinetics and efficacy of rectal versus oral sustained release morphine in cancer patients. *Cancer Chemother Pharmacol.* 1992;31:251-254.

Evaluation and Management of Emergent Conditions

Common Emergent Conditions

Early in their training, healthcare professionals are conditioned to respond quickly to emergencies, such as chest pain that may indicate myocardial infarction or breathing problems that may signal an exacerbation of chronic obstructive pulmonary disease. In emergencies, time matters and the patient is at risk of serious morbidity or death.

Cancer patients are prone to several urgent situations during which prompt diagnosis and rapid treatment may prolong life or prevent functional loss. Common emergent conditions include hypercalcemia, spinal cord compression, and obstructions of the superior vena cava, bilateral ureteral, or bowel. New onset seizure activity and hemorrhage also are frightening for patients and family members, and require immediate attention. Regardless of diagnosis, other compelling symptoms requiring urgent assessments and interventions include intractable pain, intractable emesis, severe dyspnea, and anxiety/panic attacks, all of which are covered in other modules.

In hospice and palliative care settings, emergencies may require diagnostics and interventional treatments of the underlying problem, particularly early in the course of a terminal illness when the patient's quality of life is acceptable and the likelihood of regaining prior functional levels is high. Later in the illness trajectory, specific therapies to correct underlying problems may only prolong the dying process and pose undue burdens on patients and families. In such cases, more appropriate responses include ensuring patient comfort and relieving the patient's and family's anxiety about future suffering.

Hypercalcemia

Hypercalcemia is one of the most common and difficult oncologic emergencies to diagnose because its symptoms are variable, and mimic those of advanced cancers, other advanced diseases, and the dying process itself. When onset is insidious, hypercalcemia may be confused with uncontrolled diabetes mellitus, hepatic metastases, opioid-induced side effects, or tumor invasion of the central nervous system.

Hypercalcemia should be suspected in patients with multiple myeloma and in patients with breast, lung, and kidney cancer, particularly when bone metastases are present. Symptoms of hypercalcemia include polyuria, polydipsia, fatigue, muscle weakness, anorexia, nausea, constipation, and abdominal pain. In severe cases, symptoms also include confusion, lethargy, and even coma. Electrocardiographic abnormalities and cardiac arrhythmias also can occur. A diagnosis of hypercalcemia is confirmed by an elevated serum calcium level (when corrected for an abnormal albumen, if present). Serum electrolytes and renal function must be assessed if calcium is elevated and treatment is desired.

When treatment goals include prolonging life so patients can return to a previously acceptable quality of life or undergo treatment for an underlying cancer, severe or new onset hypercalcemia may require inpatient admission. Rapid hydration with normal saline to correct dehydration and force calciuresis is the initial step. Pharmaceutical options range from relatively weak agents, such as phosphosoda and glucocorticoids, to stronger agents, such as plicamycin, calcitonin, pamidronate, and gallium nitrate. Each has advantages and disadvantages. Biphosphanates such as pamidronate are considered the treatment of choice for severe hypercalcemia. It is administered in a single 60-90 mg intravenous dose, which returns serum calcium to normal in 80 percent to 100 percent of patients, for weeks or months at a time. Pamidronate is a potent inhibitor of osteoclast-mediated skeletal resorption but does not cause mineralization defects, though its onset of action is delayed for 1 to 2 days. Calcitonin acts within minutes of administration through receptors on osteoclasts, thus decreasing the release of skeletal calcium, phosphorous, and hydroxyproline. When hypercalcemia is life-threatening, calcitonin can be administered while waiting for more sustained effects from agents such as biphosphonates or plicamycin.

In some situations, the most appropriate and humane response may be to withhold treatment of hypercalcemia. When treatment will only return patients to a chronic state of symptomatic illness with recurring hypercalcemia, patients may choose death from hypercalcemia rather than continued treatments, which may only subject them to death from other, more troublesome causes. When patients choose comfort care only, treatment focuses on effective management of pain, dehydration, nausea, constipation, and delirium. Compassionate explanations of the likely causes of hypercalcemia, its symptoms,

and the benefits and burdens of treatment options can be very reassuring for patients and families, and can help them make more informed decisions.

Spinal Cord Compression

Spinal cord compression is challenging because its most common early symptom—back pain—occurs frequently in cancer patients. Hospice and palliative medicine physicians should maintain a high index of suspicion for spinal cord compression and treat it as soon as possible to preserve patient function as much as possible. Once cord compression progresses to weakness in the lower extremities, restoring the patient's ability to walk may be difficult or impossible. Conscientious serial neurologic exams should be performed immediately when cord compression is suspected. Localized paraspinal or referred pain are common, early symptoms. When these symptoms are accompanied by radicular neuropathy, a change in gait, numbness, urinary retention, incontinence, or new constipation, suspicion should be heightened. An area of abnormality on plain films increases the likelihood of this diagnosis. Appropriate diagnostic imaging includes MRI or, if MRI is not readily available, CT myelography or routine plain myelography.

Once suspected or diagnosed, treatment with dexamethasone in doses of at least 4-8 mg qid is indicated. Bed rest may be required when the patient's spine is unstable. Prompt consultation with a radiation oncologist and possibly a neurosurgeon is recommended. When cord compression is secondary to an underlying cancer, radiation therapy is the most appropriate first-line treatment. Surgery is indicated when no previous tissue diagnosis exists or when compression recurs in a previously radiated area. Surgery should also be considered when neurologic progression occurs during radiation treatments.

For ambulatory patients with a life expectancy of a few weeks to months, pursuing a diagnosis and providing treatment are appropriate choices if they can be tolerated by the patient. The alternative to treatment is progression to paraplegia, an indwelling Foley catheter, constipation due to lack of rectal sensation, and high risk for decubitus ulcers. Bed-bound patients are unlikely to benefit from evaluation because treatment will not improve the patient's quality of life and may result only in unnecessary disruption and discomfort. In either case, establishing a bowel regimen and focusing on bladder care, pain management, and skin care are most important. As with hypercalcemia, both patients and family members benefit from compassionate education and discussion of options.

Superior Vena Cava Obstruction

Although superior vena cava obstruction generally is not life-threatening and its onset is often gradual, it is considered an oncologic emergency. Superior vena cava obstruction can be very frightening for patients and may be disfiguring. Obstruction results from tumor growth in the right, upper mediastinum and is most often associated with lung cancer, though it can occur with lymphomas or metastatic cancers to the lung. Direct observation may reveal facial plethora and facial and upper extremity edema. Swelling is aggravated by recumbence and may diminish after sitting or standing. Other symptoms include hoarseness due to vocal cord edema, headache from cerebral edema, cough, and shortness of breath. Key physical findings include dilated collateral veins over the chest wall and distention of arm veins that is unrelieved when the arms are raised above head level. Dyspnea and stridor indicate the need for urgent intervention.

Evaluation beyond physical examination includes chest x-ray with confirmation of the diagnosis by Doppler venography, CT scanning, bilateral upper extremity nuclear, or contrast venography. Initial symptomatic treatment consists of simple elevation of the head and avoidance of venipunctures and IV access in the upper extremities. Diuretics offer minimal benefit and the use of dexamethasone is controversial; however, the latter may reduce edema and permit improved flow, especially in the case of lymphoma. When the underlying cancer is chemo-sensitive and the patient is "chemo-naïve," definitive treatment is chemotherapy. When the tumor is less chemo-sensitive or the patient has received extensive previous treatment, radiation therapy is the preferred treatment.

Occasionally, superior vena cava obstruction recurs after definitive radiation. Then, education and treatment of distressing symptoms are the most appropriate choices. For example, positioning is important for relieving associated dyspnea. Education and treatment also are appropriate when superior vena cava obstruction occurs in an otherwise debilitated patient who cannot tolerate or does not desire specific diagnostic or therapeutic interventions.

Cardiac Tamponade

Cardiac tamponade occurs when increases in pericardial fluid or stiffening of the pericardial sac prevent adequate right heart filling and left heart pumping, leading to decreased cardiac output with resultant hypotension and dyspnea. One of the most common causes of cardiac tamponade is tumor spread to the lungs or mediastinum. Pericardial involvement occurs most commonly with lung and breast cancers, lymphomas, and leukemias. Rarely is it caused by previous mediastinal radiation therapy.

Patients usually complain of chest pain, dyspnea, cough, orthopnea, weakness, and dizziness. Physical exam may reveal pulsus paradoxicus, hypotension, muffled heart sounds, a friction rub, or tachycardia. A diagnosis of cardiac tamponade should be suspected when chest radiography reveals new cardiomegaly, or when electrocardiograms indicate low QRS voltage or electrical alternans. Echocardiography documents the presence of pericardial fluid and evaluates heart function.

Pericardiocentesis provides rapid relief of tamponade. To prevent the return of fluid, it may be necessary to perform a pericardial window procedure or drain the space with a catheter and instill a sclerosing agent. When the patient is very near death, is not a surgical candidate, or does not desire invasive interventions, treatment focuses on symptom control with analgesics, anxiolytics, and oxygen. In any case, compassionate education and assurances of continued care for the patient should be provided.

Urinary Obstruction

Urinary obstruction usually presents insidiously. The patient may not be aware of a decline in urine output or may present with an inability to void. Other symptoms may include abdominal discomfort, malaise, and nausea.

Ureteral obstruction occurs most commonly with pelvic cancers or cancers involving the retroperitoneal lymph nodes, such as cancers of the prostate, cervix, rectum, and lymphomas. Serum chemistries reveal elevated serum creatinine and blood urea nitrogen, and possibly electrolyte abnormalities. Bladder outlet obstruction is common and must be ruled out with Foley catheterization. The best diagnostic test is renal ultrasound. The principal finding is unilateral or bilateral dilatation of the renal pelvis.

Treatment starts with relieving pain and nausea and determining the patient's goals of therapy, if possible. Renal failure can be a relatively painless cause of death. Relieving ureteral obstruction with internal ureteral stents or external nephrostomy drainage usually leads to improved renal function and can be life-prolonging. However, external urinary drainage may be unacceptable to some patients, nephrostomies are prone to infection as well as occasional leakage and

blockage, and drainage may not be appropriate for patients who are near death or whose quality of life is poor. In such cases, antiemetics and other symptomatic treatments may be more appropriate and humane.

Bowel Obstruction

Malignant bowel obstruction occurs in 3 percent of all terminally ill cancer patients, most commonly in patients with colorectal and ovarian cancer. Obstruction also occurs in patients with endometrial, gastric, mesothelial, and prostatic malignancies. Pathophysiologic mechanisms causing bowel obstruction include: (1) extrinsic compression of the lumen; (2) intraluminal occlusion of the lumen; (3) intramural occlusion of the lumen; (4) intestinal motility disorders; and (5) other miscellaneous causes such as fecal impaction, inflammatory edema, or medications that cause severe constipation. Symptoms may vary according to the level of obstruction, but diagnosis is typically straightforward when patients present with characteristic symptoms of intestinal colic, abdominal pain, and nausea or vomiting.

Appropriate treatment of bowel obstruction depends on the patient's estimated life expectancy. Surgery may be an appropriate option when patients have an extended life expectancy and both the patient and physician agree that surgery offers significant benefit. The placement of a venting gastrostomy tube may relieve the discomfort of high intestinal obstructions and facilitate mechanical decompression of the bowel. When patients are near death, symptomatic treatment is more appropriate and should focus on relief of three primary symptoms: intestinal colic, abdominal pain, and nausea or vomiting. Anticholinergics inhibit spasmodic activity that causes the paroxysms of intestinal colic and should be used generously. Abdominal pain can also be relieved with strong opioids. Nausea and vomiting can be controlled with combinations of antiemetics, corticosteroids, and octreotide.

Corticosteroids decrease peritumor edema, and their use may actually decrease the obstructive process itself. Octreotide, a somatostatin analog, greatly diminishes gastrointestinal secretions and motility, and reduces splanchnic blood flow, thus decreasing abdominal distention, vomiting, and pain. In hospice and palliative care settings, nasogastric tubes are not commonly used to control the symptoms of bowel obstruction—they are uncomfortable and rarely necessary.

Hemorrhage

Hemorrhage can be very frightening for patients and family members. It may occur suddenly, leaving no time for a home visit or for transporting the patient to an inpatient setting. The most effective plan is to anticipate bleeding, educate the patient and family about appropriate responses, and provide ongoing emotional support.

Bleeding may be secondary to underlying defects in the clotting system. It may also result from ulcers of the gastrointestinal tract or skin, or tumor erosion of blood vessels. In patients with leukemias, multiple myeloma, or myelodysplasia, thrombocytopenia may lead to hemorrhage. Thrombocytopenia also may occur after intense chemotherapy or when solid tumors replace bone marrow, for example, in breast cancer, lymphoma, or prostate cancer. Coagulopathies also may result in hemorrhage, for example, cancer-related disseminated intravascular coagulation (DIC). Patients with liver failure from cirrhosis may experience insufficient production of clotting proteins. Patients receiving long-term anticoagulation therapy are likely to experience increased clotting times when their oral intake decreases and their metabolism slows. Such patients often require dosage adjustments or complete cessation of anticoagulation therapy when the primary goal of treatment changes from cure to comfort.

Mechanical causes of rapid bleeding are associated with tumors located near numerous small blood vessels, for example, in stomach or rectal cancers, or when tumors are located near large vessels, for example, head and neck cancers adjacent to the carotids. Occasionally, external bleeding is related to ulcerated tumors of the breast. Patients may develop upper gastrointestinal bleeding due to stress, peptic ulcers, or treatment with steroids or NSAIDs. Endobronchial tumors can result in small but frightening hemoptysis or massive, terminal hemoptysis. The likelihood of small hemoptysis is reduced with the use of antitussive therapy, for example, codeine. Massive hemoptyis may cause dyspnea, anxiety, and overwhelming fright in patients and family members.

As with other emergent situations, appropriate interventions depend on the patient's prior status and ability to tolerate a procedure, and the goals of treatment. Interventions may prolong good quality of life or merely extend the dying process. As always, the primary goal is immediate patient comfort and reduction of anxiety and fear. Additional interventions may include factor replacement, surgery, or other treatments.

When bleeding is probable, anticipatory measures are required, including patient and family education, timely review of appropriate responses to emergencies, and ready access to on-call health professionals, for example, a hospice home care team. A supply of non-sterile gloves and dark towels should be kept nearby to absorb blood and help disguise the amount of blood loss. Anxiolytics should be readily available, preferably in oral, sublingual, rectal, or even parenteral formulations. Most family members can be trained to administer anxiolytics rectally and parenterally, if needed.

Seizures

New-onset seizures are likely to be extremely frightening for patients and family members. Differential diagnosis includes metabolic abnormalities such as hypoglycemia, alcohol withdrawal, cardiac arrhythmias, and (most commonly in cancer patients) brain metastases. As in other emergent situations, the first step is to ensure the patient's comfort, then, if possible, to determine the patient's and family's wishes regarding further diagnostic evaluation and goals of treatment. If the patient does not want or cannot tolerate radiation therapy, or has previously received whole brain radiation, diagnostic evaluations other than a bedside neurological exam are unwarranted.

Because seizures are so frightening to witness, impair the patient's functional status and level of alertness, and contribute to safety concerns, they should be treated acutely.

Medication should be used to relieve seizing and prevent further seizures. When the patient is actively seizing, parenteral lorazepam or diazepam should be administered. Once the patient is stable, anti-convulsant treatment should begin with loading doses of phenytoin followed by routine administration. When patients cannot swallow, or lose the ability to swallow, phenobarbital can be administered in rectal form or with a single daily injection.

Other emergent situations that require immediate attention and rapid therapeutic intervention include delirium, rapid escalation of pain, severe dyspnea, intractable nausea, and vomiting. These topics are covered in other modules.

Objectives

Attitudes/Behaviors

1. Identify goals and values that are likely to influence a terminally ill patient's choice of treatments for common emergencies.

2. Explain why treatment options are not uniformly applicable to all patients.

3. Discuss the potential for conflicting treatment goals among patients and family members.

4. Describe potential benefits and burdens of various diagnostic and treatment options for patients and families.

5. Justify the provision of symptomatic palliative therapy whether or not treatment is directed at the underlying cause of an emergency.

6. Defend the withholding of specific standard therapies when a patient's treatment goal changes from prolonging life to comfort care only.

7. Defend the acceptance of an uncertain diagnosis when a patient's treatment goal is comfort only.

8. Explain appropriate responses to emergent situations that are particularly frightening for terminally ill patients and their family members.

9. Describe specific scenarios in which an underlying condition should not be treated when a terminally ill patient is experiencing an emergent symptom.

10. Discuss the need for rapid treatment of spinal cord compression in ambulatory terminally ill patients with a life expectancy of weeks to months.

Knowledge

1. Discuss common clinical scenarios in which the following medical emergencies are experienced by patients with advanced disease: hypercalcemia, spinal cord compression, superior vena cava obstruction, urinary obstruction, bowel obstruction, cardiac tamponade, bleeding, and new-onset seizures.

2. Explain common signs and symptoms of the following oncologic emergencies: hypercalcemia, spinal cord compression, superior vena cava obstruction, urinary obstruction, bowel obstruction, and cardiac tamponade.

3. Describe potential causes of acute onset seizures.

4. Describe appropriate diagnostic strategies for: hypercalcemia, spinal cord compression, superior vena cava obstruction, cardiac tamponade, bowel obstruction, and urinary obstruction.

5. Describe the standard treatments for each of the previously mentioned emergencies.

6. Explain the standard pharmacologic management of hypercalcemia.

7. Discuss the pharmacologic management of seizures.

8. Discuss potential differences in treatment based on the patient's condition and setting in the following clinical scenarios: hypercalcemia, seizures, and spinal cord compression,

9. Discuss the use of nasogastric tubes when treating bowel obstruction in patients in hospice and palliative care settings.

10. Describe various pharmaceuticals used to treat symptoms associated with bowel obstruction.

Skills

1. Explain to patients and family members the differential diagnoses and treatment options for the previously mentioned emergencies.

2. Help patients and family members determine goals of treatment based on the patient's values and goals, as well as the clinical scenario and setting.

3. Demonstrate appropriate pharmacologic treatment of hypercalcemia.

4. Evaluate a patient with possible spinal cord compression appropriately.

5. Collaborate with surgical subspecialists and radiation oncologists when determining appropriate treatments for patients with spinal cord compression, superior vena cava syndrome, or cardiac tamponade.

6. Effectively treat the symptoms caused by the previously described emergencies.

7. Prepare a patient's family to cope with potential massive hemorrhage.

8. Prescribe anticonvulsants for patients who can swallow and for those who have lost the ability to swallow.

References

1. Abner A. Approach to the patient who presents with superior vena cava obstruction. *Chest.* 1993;103:394s-397s. (suppl 4)

2. Bajorunas DR. Clinical manifestations of cancer-related hypercalcemia. *Semin Oncol.* 1990;17(2):16-25. (suppl 5)

3. Berger A, Portenoy RK, Weissman DE, eds. *Principles and Practice of Supportive Oncology.* Philadelphia: Lippincott-Raven; 1998.

4. Bilezikian JP. Management of acute hypercalcemia. *New Engl J Med.* 1992; 326(18): 1196-1203.

5. DeVita VT, Hellman S, Rosenberg SA, eds. *Cancer: Principles and Practice of Oncology.* 5th edition. Philadelphia: J.B. Lippincott Co.; 1997.

6. Hicks F, Thom V, Alison D, Corcoran G. Spinal cord compression: the hospice perspective. *J Palliat Care.* 1994;9(3):9-13.

7. Ingham J, Beveridge A, Cooney NJ. The management of spinal cord compression in patient with advanced malignancy. *J Pain Symptom Manage.* 1993; 8(1):1-6.

8. Markman M. Common complications and emergencies associated with cancer and its therapy. *Cleve Clin J Med.* 1994; 61(2):105-14.

9. Mundy GR, Martin TJ. Hypercalcemia of malignancy: pathogenesis and management. *Metabolism.* 1992; 31:1247-1277.

10. Ralston SH, Gallacher SJ, Patel U., et al. Cancer-associated hypercalcemia: morbidity and mortality. Clinical experience in 126 treated patients. *Ann Intern Med.* 1990;112(7): 499-504.

11. Rousseau, P. Nonpain symptom management in terminal care. *Clin Geriatric Med.* 1996; 12(2):313-327.

12. Sherrard DJ. Letter: Do everything you can. *Ann Intern Med.* 1990;113(1):84.

13. Smith J. Oncologic emergencies. In: Patt R, ed. *Cancer Pain.* Philadelphia: J.B. Lippincott; 1993:527-542.

14. Twycross RG, Lack SA. *Therapeutics in Terminal Cancer.* London: Pitman Publishing, Ltd., 1984.

15. Yellin A, Rosen A, Reichert N, et al. Superior vena cava syndrome: the myth—the facts. *Am Rev Respir Dis.* 1990;141(5): 1114-1118.

Evaluation and Management of General Non-Pain Symptoms

Anorexia

Because good nutrition plays a vital role in maintaining quality of life, most cultures view the provision of food and water as a means of showing love, respect, nurturing, and caring. However, loss of appetite is common in cancer and other end-stage diseases. As disease advances, most terminally ill patients consume progressively smaller amounts of food and fluid. Caregivers may view the patient's rejection of food as a symbolic personal rejection, thus patient and family education plays an important role in the management of anorexia. Common causes of loss of appetite include:

- Drugs and therapies, such as chemotherapy and radiation
- Pain, fatigue, anxiety, depression, fear of vomiting, aversion to food (sight, odors, temperatures, and textures), and attempts to eat too much food
- Biochemical causes, such as hypokalemia, hyponatremia, hyper or hypoglycemia, uremia, hypercalcemia, and underlying infection
- Gastrointestinal involvement, such as infection, ulceration, autonomic dysfunction, obstruction, or constipation
- Malodorous ulcers
- Cancer itself and some tumor products such as tumor necrosis factor (TNF) and interleukin 1 (IL-1)

Although anorexia often is a normal symptom of far-advanced disease, treatment is indicated if anorexia distresses the patient. When possible, treatment is aimed at underlying causes. Management techniques include:

- Offering small, frequent, visually attractive meals of the patient's favorite foods at room temperature or cold (Former dietary restrictions can be discontinued.)
- Using appetite stimulants, such as small amounts of alcohol before meals, cyproheptadine, prokinetic drugs (metoclopramide, cisapride), corticosteroids (prednisone, dexamethasone), progestins (megestrol acetate), or cannabinoids (dronabinol)

Enteral Feeding

Enteral feeding requires placement of a nasogastric, gastrostomy, or jejunostomy tube. Tube feedings and forced feeding have never been shown to increase survival in terminally ill cancer patients. They can predispose the patient to reflux and aspiration pneumonia and can lead to fluid overload, increased secretions, and diarrhea. Enteral feeding may be helpful for patients with head and neck or esophageal tumors who are unable to swallow and still have an appetite. They may also be useful for patients with neurological swallowing disorders who can reasonably be expected to maintain functional status and to experience improved quality of life with improved nutrition. However, treatment with enteral nutritional therapy must be individualized and should focus on symptom relief. As the patient's condition changes, the relative benefits and burdens of tube feedings should be reassessed frequently.

Total parenteral nutrition (TPN) is rarely used in hospice/palliative care settings. It is generally not effective in improving a patient's survival or response to anti-cancer therapy. In fact, a meta-analysis of 12 trials showed TPN resulted in decreased survival, a decreased response to chemotherapy, and increased rates of infection. However, TPN has been shown to increase weight gain and improve quality of life in selected patients with HIV disease. As always, therapy should be individualized, with careful consideration of the benefits and burdens of treatment.

Cachexia

Cachexia is the end result of a number of advanced diseases and may be associated with anorexia, chronic nausea, asthenia, and changes in body image. Causes of cachexia include malnutrition due to poor intake, obstruction, malabsorption, protein loss, gastrointestinal loss, and tumor burden. Cachexia is not reversed by intensive nutritional therapy, and is often accompanied by anxiety and depression on the part of the patient, the family, and caregivers. Helping patients and family members focus on alternative ways of expressing caring is increasingly important as the disease progresses and the burdens of treating anorexia begin to outweigh its benefits.

Dehydration

During the end stages of disease, patients often consume less fluid due to increased frailty, a decreased sense of thirst, reduced levels of consciousness, and the effects of

sedative and antimuscarinic drugs often used to palliate other symptoms. Dehydration is exacerbated by fluid loss due to vomiting and diarrhea. Typically, as patients near the end of life, they do not experience the classic symptoms of dehydration, which include thirst, dry mouth, dysphagia, apathy, depression, headache, muscle cramps, and, if sweating is impaired, pyrexia. Dehydration may actually relieve intracranial pressure and reduce the edema surrounding tumors, resulting in decreased pain.

Some healthcare professionals believe dehydration contributes to a painful and distressing death due to electrolyte imbalances that result in agitation, disorientation, and neuromuscular irritability. They argue that hydration can prevent constipation, decubiti, and renal failure and terminal confusion, possibly as a result of increased excretion of toxic metabolites. Hypodermoclysis (subcutaneous administration of fluids) can be used to administer fluids, either continuously or by bolus, with the addition of hyaluronidase to facilitate absorption. Small needles prevent discomfort and intravenous catheterization is avoided.

Other professionals believe artificial hydration offers no proven benefits and may impose additional physical and psychological burdens on patients and caregivers. They argue that artificial hydration can increase pharyngeal and pulmonary secretions, which results in the need for increased suctioning, sensations of choking and nausea, and vomiting. Artificial hydration may also exacerbate symptoms of cardiac, renal, or hepatic failure, and lead to increased urine output, with increased discomfort to the patient and burden to the caregivers. Because the patient's sense of thirst is relieved with ice chips and sips of fluid in amounts less than those necessary to alleviate thirst due to dehydration in non-terminal patients, opponents of artificial hydration also argue that sensations of thirst in the terminally ill population are unrelated to electrolyte abnormalities or rates of fluid administration.

The administration of enteral, intravenous or subcutaneous fluids remains controversial. As with any treatment, the primary goal is increasing the patient's comfort. Food and fluids requested by patients should be provided; however, the administration of fluids beyond those needed to relieve symptoms of thirst and dry mouth may not be consistent with the principles of palliative care. As with any treatment, the burdens and benefits of artificial hydration should be carefully considered from the patient's point of view.

Asthenia

Asthenia is one of the most prevalent symptoms in patients with advanced cancer. It frequently coexists with anorexia and malnutrition, is characterized by fatigue, low energy, and generalized weakness, and is sometimes accompanied by weight loss and decreased muscle bulk and function. Causes of weakness include:

- Nerve or muscle damage or the side effects of surgery, chemotherapy, or radiation
- Myasthenic syndrome (Eaton-Lambert), paraneoplastic process, electrolyte imbalance (Na, K, Ca, P04), dehydration, and organ failure
- Drugs such as opioids, sedatives, antidepressants, antihypertensives, antiarrythmics, and diuretics

When possible, treatment of weakness is aimed at underlying causes such as anemia, electrolyte imbalance, dehydration, or fever. Weakness due to neuromyopathy may respond to a trial of corticosteroids; however, long-term use may induce proximal myopathy of the extremities. Weakness due to insomnia and depression should be treated with appropriate pharmacological and non-pharmacological interventions. Weakness due to prolonged immobility may be helped with:

- Improved symptom control and mobilization, which can increase the patient's range of motion
- Physical therapy, which may improve the patient's functional status and add to patient satisfaction
- Massage, passive exercises, and use of a hospital bed with an overhead trapeze which may provide support and mobilization for weak patients

As weakness progresses, it is important to take time to discuss with patients, family members, and caregivers the psychological and spiritual issues commonly associated with generalized deterioration.

Fever

Fever in patients with cancer may be due to an inflammatory response triggered by tumor cells or by the release of pyrogens from tumor cells. Fever can occur with any tumor type but is most often associated with lymphomas and leukemias, myelodysplastic syndromes, renal cell carcinoma, hepatoma, and atrial myxoma. Infections that produce fever may be related to the tumor, for example, post-obstructive pneumonia, or unrelated, for example, urinary tract infection or pulmonary embolus. Drug reactions and anti-cancer therapies such as cytokine and radiation therapy can also produce fever.

Fever may not occur during the end stages of disease or it may be suppressed by concurrent therapy or present atypically. Searching for the underlying cause of fever may be warranted if improvements in the patient's quality of life are likely to result from specific therapy aimed at the cause. Antibiotic therapy can be started empirically while awaiting test results, but antibiotics should not be used as antipyretics. In hospice/palliative care settings, antibiotics are most often used to relieve distressing symptoms such as painful dysuria, cough, dyspnea, painful wounds, infectious diarrhea, foul-smelling necrotic tumors, or dysphagia from candidiasis. Decisions to initiate antibiotic therapy to prolong life should be individualized, for example, when the patient wants to live long enough to see a new grandchild. When treatment of the underlying cause of the fever is not consistent with the patient's goals for therapy and the administration of antibiotics would serve only to prolong the process of dying, palliative therapies should be used. They include treatment with antipyretics (including nonsteroidal anti-inflammatory agents and acetaminophen, many of which are available in liquid form), other medications to palliate distressing symptoms, and local measures to improve comfort. Aggressive medical treatment of infections in patients with end-stage Alzheimer's disease has limited effect on length of life.

Sleep Disturbances

Sleep disturbances may result from single or multiple etiologies. The following factors should be considered:

- Physical discomfort
- Medication effects, including withdrawal
- Metabolic abnormalities; the abnormalities that produce anorexia can also lead to sleeplessness
- Organ failure and increased intracranial pressure, which may cause generalized restlessness and insomnia
- Emotional contributors such as fear, anger, guilt, and spiritual concerns

Often, an interdisciplinary approach is required to relieve sleep disturbances. Comprehensive interventions include counseling, education, imagery, massage, breathing exercises, progressive relaxation, and use of hypnotic agents if necessary. Medications should be individualized but typically include a short-acting benzodiazepine or an antihistamine.

Myoclonus

Multifocal myoclonus may occur in patients being treated with high doses of opioids, in particular morphine. Because reductions in the opioid dose are likely to result in the return of pain, it is usually necessary to switch to a different opioid (opioid rotation) or add a benzodiazepine.

Terminal Restlessness

Restlessness with or without confusion and/or agitation may occur during the final hours or days of a person's life and can be very distressing for the patient, family, and caregivers. Symptoms include repetitive behavior, increased movement, confusion, paranoia, hallucinations, nightmares, insomnia, and dyspnea, with lengthening periods of drowsiness or exhaustion. Treatment is directed at maintaining a calm, supportive environment and providing ongoing reassurance for the patient and caregivers. Sedative medications may be necessary to relieve symptoms and can include a benzodiazepine, an antipsychotic, or a barbiturate. The medications can be used in combination and may be administered by a variety of routes, for example, orally, parenterally, subcutaneously, or rectally.

Pruritus

Pruritus is common in those patients with cholestasis, uremia, lymphoma, myeloproliferative disorders, iron deficiency, carcinomatosis, intraspinal morphine, endocrine disorders, and dry skin. Treatment is aimed at the underlying cause and can include surgical bypass of a biliary obstruction, stent placement, and other therapeutic interventions such as the addition of a bile resin binder for pruritus due to hepatic disorders. Myeloproliferative disorders may respond to a trial of NSAIDs or to an H2 blocker.

Although commonly associated with antibiotic therapy, pruritus can result from any drug. A careful review of medications may suggest an etiology, with discontinuation of the offending agent being the treatment of choice. Local therapy, such as a tepid water bath with colloidal oatmeal, not soap, may be indicated. Emollients, or oils, for dry skin can be used liberally. Effective topical therapies include calamine lotion, menthol or topical anesthetic agents, and corticosteroids. Antihistamine medications (hydroxyzine, diphenhydramine) may provide some relief but often are sedating. Phenothiazines (promethazine, chlorpromazine) have good antihistamine and antipruritic effects, although they can also be sedating and have anticholinergic side effects. Hydroxyzine has sedative effects in addition to antihistamine and anxiolytic effects, and may have analgesic action as well. Cyproheptadine and pizotifen have antihistamine and antiserotonin action. Anxiolytics (e.g. benzodiazepines) may improve pruritus. Corticosteroids used topically and/or systemically may be effective in the treatment of pruritus due to cholestasis or lymphoproliferative disorders. Transcutaneous electrical nerve stimulation, capsaicin cream, physical therapy, and distraction techniques can be helpful.

Fungating and Ulcerating Tumors

Fungation occurs most commonly with tumors of the head, neck, and breast, and can result in distressing disfigurement, pain, and odor. Treatments include radiation therapy and/or chemotherapy for sensitive tumors. In some cases, surgery may be warranted. Local care includes cleansing with normal saline or water and frequent dressing changes using non-adherent, absorptive dressings. Alginate dressings can help prevent bleeding during dressing changes and can absorb exudate. Metronidazole gel and topical antibiotics may control infection and reduce odor. Charcoal or chloresium dressings can also reduce odor. Systemic antibiotic therapy with anaerobic coverage may help control infection, odor, and pain in some settings.

Decubiti (Pressure Sores)

Pressure sores commonly occur in terminally ill patients. The following conditions contribute to their formation:

- Immobility, weakness, debility, poor nutrition, loss of subcutaneous tissue, moisture, irritants, and incontinence
- Pressure, friction (dragging a patient across sheets), and shear forces (sliding down in the bed when the head of the bed is at an angle)
- Corticosteroid therapy, chemotherapy, radiation, sedation, altered mental status, contractures, dementia, ascites, and analgesics

Therapy is indicated by the grade of the pressure sore but secondary infections can complicate care.

- Grade 1 sores are characterized by blanchable erythema
- Grade 2 sores are characterized by an area of non-blanchable erythema and can include excoriation, vesiculation, or skin breakdown of the epidermis
- Grade 3 sores involve drainage and full thickness skin loss, but not loss of subcutaneous tissue
- Grade 4 sores extend into subcutaneous fat and deep fascia, with possible muscle and bone involvement

Ulcers may be cleaned with normal saline or a commercial preparation but caustic agents such as iodine, hydrogen peroxide, and sodium hypochlorite should be avoided. Grade 1-3 ulcers may be dressed and protected with a hydrocolloid dressing such as duoderm or comfeel. Calcium alginate dressings can be useful for exudative wounds. Necrotic tissue and eschar can be removed or debrided with agents such as collagenase or elase, or by the proper use of debriding dressings. Systemic antibiotics may be useful if there is evidence of cellulitis or osteomyelitis.

Ideally, pressure sores can be prevented by identifying patients at risk and implementing the following measures to aid healing and prevent further skin breakdown:

- Keeping skin clean, dry, and moisturized
- Using a commercial cleaning agent and moisture barrier

- Reducing shear forces by using sheepskin and drawsheets for lifting patients
- Repositioning frequently, e.g., every 2-4 hours
- Using specially designed beds, mattresses, and dressings

When managing pressure sores, the goals of therapy should be guided by the patient's condition and probable length of life. Even with scrupulous care, pressure sores are sometimes inevitable in terminally ill patients. Patients, family members, and caregivers should be reassured that pressure sores do not automatically indicate inadequate care.

Objectives

Attitudes/Behaviors

1. Defend the provision or withdrawal of nutritional support in a hospice or palliative care setting.

2. Defend the provision or withdrawal of artificial hydration in a hospice or palliative care setting.

3. Differentiate among the goals of the physician, patient, and caregiver in the provision of palliative care.

4. Initiate a care plan which is guided by the philosophy and values of the patient for the symptoms given.

5. Discuss how various treatment options for each symptom might affect the patient and family.

6. Discuss the impact of cultural and religious backgrounds on the patient and family treatment preferences.

7. Identify your own treatment biases and how they impact your delivery of care.

8. Compare the potential meaning of the symptom complex for the patient, physician, and caregiver.

9. Explain the importance of the various members of the interdisciplinary team in providing comfort care for each of the symptom complexes.

Knowledge

1. Propose a diagnostic plan for each of the symptom complexes given in this module.

2. Identify the potential burdens and benefits of treating each of the symptom complexes given.

3. Describe non-pharmacological methods for addressing each of the symptom complexes listed.

4. Discuss the available medications, dosages, routes, advantages, and disadvantages of pharmacotherapy for each symptom complex.

5. Describe indications for selection, contraindications, alternatives, side effects, toxicity, method of action, potential interactions, and cost of treatments for specific symptoms.

6. Discuss the various settings where the symptom complexes may be encountered (home, hospital, clinic, nursing home) and how their treatment will be affected by the setting.

7. Discuss the economic issues surrounding treatment options for the symptom complexes.

8. Describe the different grades of decubitus ulcers.

9. Describe the treatments for each grade of decubitus ulcers.

Skills

1. Collaborate with the interdisciplinary team and provide specific information about diseases, symptom complexes, diagnostic processes, medical management, and symptom control.

2. Utilize the interdisciplinary team for comprehensive symptom control.

3. Communicate with the patient, family, and/or caregiver about symptom management.

4. Provide guidance for patients and family members as they make the transition from focusing on cure and health maintenance to providing comfort and symptom relief.

5. Make decisions using patient input to maximize patient control.

6. Utilize multidimensional assessments including medical, psychological, social, emotional, spiritual, and functional, for each symptom used in this module.

7. Treat various stages of decubitus ulcers effectively.

References

1. Andrews M, Bell ER, Smith SA, Tischier JF, Veglia JM. Dehydration in terminally ill patients: is it appropriate palliative care? *Postgrad Med*. 1993;93(1):201-3; 206-8.
2. Anorexia. In: *Medical Care of the Dying*. Victoria, British Columbia: Victoria Hospice Society; 1993:250.
3. Berger EY. Nutrition by hypodermoclysis. *J Am Geriatr Soc*. 1984;32:199-203.
4. Billings JA. Comfort measures for the terminally ill: is dehydration painful? *J Am Geriatr Soc*. 1985;33(11):808-810.
5. Billings JA. Anorexia. *J Palliat Care*. 1994;10(1):51-3.

6. Boyd KJ, Beeken L. Tube feeding in palliative care: benefits and problems. *Palliat Med*. 1994;8:156-158.

7. Bruera E, de Stoutz ND, Fainsinger RL, Spachynski K, Suarez-Almazor M, Hanson J. Comparison of two different concentrations of hyaluronidase in patients receiving one hour infusions of hypodermoclysis. *J Pain Symptom Manage*. 1995;10(7):505-509.

8. Bruera E, Fainsinger RL: Clinical management of cachexia and anorexia. In: *Oxford Textbook of Palliative Medicine*, Doyle D, Hanks GW, and MacDonald N, eds. New York: Oxford University Press; 1993:330-337.

9. Bruera E, Franco JJ, Maltoni M, Watanabe S, Suarez-Almazor M. Changing pattern of agitated impaired mental status in patients with advanced cancer: association with cognitive monitoring, hydration, and opioid rotation. *J Pain Symptom Manage*. 1995;10(4):287-291.

10. Bruera E, MacDonald RN. Asthenia in patients with advanced cancer. *J Pain Symptom Manage*. 1988; 3:9-14.

11. Bruera E, MacDonald RN. Nutrition in cancer patients: an update and review of our experience. *J Pain Symptom Manage*. 1988,3:133-140.

12. Burge GI. Dehydration symptoms of palliative care cancer patients. *J Pain Symptom Manage*. 1993;8:454-464.

13. Panel for the prediction and prevention of pressure ulcers in adults. *Pressure Ulcers in Adults: Prediction and Prevention*. Clinical Practice Guideline, Number 3, AHCPR Publication N. 92-0047. Rockville, Md: Agency of Health Care Policy and Research, Public Health Service, US Department of Health and Human Services. May 1992.

14. Coyle N, Adelhardt J, Foley KM, Portenoy RK: Character of terminal illness in the advanced cancer patient: pain and other symptoms during the last four weeks of life. *J Pain Symptom Manage*. 1990;5:83-93.

15. Craig GM. On withholding nutrition and hydration in the terminally ill: has palliative medicine gone too far? *J Med Ethics* 1994;20:139-143.

16. de Stoutz ND, Bruera E, Suarez-Almazor M. Opioid rotation for toxicity reduction in terminal cancer patients. *J Pain Symptom Manage*. 1995;10(5):378-384.

17. Dicks B. Rehydration or dehydration? *Support Care Cancer*. 1994;2(2):88-90.

18. Dunphy K, Finlay I, Rathbone G, Gilbert J, Hicks F. Rehydration in palliative and terminal care: if not- why not? *Palliat Med*. 1995; 9(3):221-228.

19. Economos K, Lucci JA, Richardson B, Yasigi R, Miller DS. The effect of naproxen on fever in patients with advanced gynecologic malignancies. *Gynecol Oncol*. 1995;56(2):250-254.

20. Ellershaw JE, Sutcliffe JM, Saunders CM. Dehydration and the dying patient. *J Pain Symptom Manage*. 1995;10(3):192-197.

21. Fainsinger R, Bruera E. The management of dehydration in terminally ill patients. *J Palliat Care*. 1994;10(3):55-59.

22. Fainsinger RL, MacEachem T, Miller MJ, et al. The use of hypodermoclysis for rehydration in terminally ill cancer patients. *J Pain Symptom Manage*. 1994;9(5):298-302.

23. Finlay IG, Bowszyc J, Ramlau C, Gwiezdzinski. The effect of topical 0.75% metronidazole gel on malodorous cutaneous ulcers. *J Pain Symptom Manage*. 1996;11(3):158-162.

24. Gillon R. Palliative care ethics: non-provision of artificial nutrition and hydration to terminally ill sedated patients. *J Med Ethics*. 1994;20:131-132,187.

25. Grauer PA. Appetite stimulants in terminal care: treatment of anorexia. *Hospice J*. 1993;9(2-3):73-83.

26. Grocott P. The palliative management of fungating malignant wounds. *J Wound Care*. 1995;4(5):240-242.

27. Hallett A. Fungating wounds. *Nurs Times*. 1995;91(39):81-82, 85.

28. Hurley AC, Volicer B, Mahoney MA, Volicer L. Palliative fever management in Alzheimer patients: quality plus fiscal responsibility. *Adv Nurs Sci*. 1993;16(l):21-32.

29. Justice D, The "natural" death while not eating: a type of palliative care in Banaras, India. *J Palliat Care*. 1995;11(1):38-42.

30. Malone N. Hydration in the terminally ill patient. *Nurs Stand*. 1994; 8(43):29-32.

31. Mecca RM, Half WJ, Groth-Juncker A. Comfort care for terminally ill patients: the appropriate use of nutrition and hydration. *JAMA*. 1994;272:1263-1266.

32. McIver B, Walsh D, Nelson K. The use of chlorpromazine for symptom control in dying cancer patients. *J Pain Symptom Manage*. 1994;9(5):341-345.

33. Meares CJ. Terminal dehydration: a review. *Am J Hospice Palliat Care*. 1994;11(3):10-14.
34. Mercadante S, DeConno F, Ripamonti C. Propofol in terminal care. *J Pain Symptom Manage*. 1995;10(8):639-642.
35. Mercadante S. Nutrition in cancer patients. *Support Care Cancer*. 1996;4(l):10-20.
36. Micetich KC, Steinecker PH, Thomasma DC. Are intravenous fluids morally required for a dying patient? *Arch Intern Med*. 1983;143:975-978.
37. Miller CM, O'Neill A, Mortimer PS. Skin problems in palliative care: nursing aspects. In: *Oxford Textbook of Palliative Medicine*. Doyle D, Hanks GW, and MacDonald N, eds. New York: Oxford University Press; 1993:395-407.
38. Morant R, Hans-Jorg S. The management of infections in palliative care. In: *Oxford Textbook of Palliative Medicine*. Doyle D, Hanks GW, and MacDonald N, eds. New York: Oxford University Press; 1993:378-384.
39. Musgrave CF, Barta. N, Opstad J, The sensation of thirst in dying patients receiving IV hydration. *J Palliat Care*. 1995;11(4):17-21.
40. Newman V, Allwood M, Oakes RA. The use of metronidazole gel to control the smell of malodorous lesions. *Palliat Med*. 1989;3:303-305.
41. Printz LA. Terminal dehydration, a compassionate treatment. *Arch Intern Med*. 1992:152(4):697-700.
42. Schonwetter RS, ed. *Clinics in Geriatric Medicine*. Care of the Terminally Ill Patient. Philadelphia: WB Saunders; 1996:12(2):237-433.
43. Sjogren P, Jonsson T, Jensen NH, Drenck NE. Staehelin JT. Hyperalgesia and myoclonus in terminal cancer patients treated with continuous intravenous morphine. *Pain*. 1993;55:93-97.
44. Sutcliffe J, Holmes S. Dehydration: burden or benefit to the dying patient? *J Adv Nurs*. 1994; 19(1):71-76.
45. Taylor MA. Benefits of dehydration in terminally ill patients. *Geriatr Nurs*. 1995;16(6):271-272.
46. Twycross RG, Lack SA. *Therapeutics in Terminal Care*. 2nd ed. Edinburgh: Churchill Livingstone; 1990.
47. Twycross RG, Lack SA. Failure to eat. In: *Therapeutics in Terminal Cancer*. Pitman Publishing Ltd; 1984:36.
48. Vigano A, Watanabe S, Bruera E. Anorexia and cachexia in advanced cancer patients. *Cancer Surv*. 1994; 21:99-115.
49. Waller A, Hershkowitz M, Adunsky A. The effect of intravenous fluid infusion on blood and urine parameters of hydration and the state of consciousness in terminal cancer patients. *Am J Hospice Palliat Care*. 1994;11(6):22-27.
50. Yan E, Bruera E. Case report: parenteral hydration of terminally ill cancer patients. *J Palliat Care*. 1991;7:40-43.
51. Yoshioka H. Rehabilitation for the terminal cancer patient. *Am J Phys Med Rehabil*. 1994;73(3):199-206.

Evaluation and Management of Cardiorespiratory Symptoms

Goal of Management

Few patients die without experiencing cardiorespiratory symptoms. As increasing numbers of patients with end-stage primary cardiac and pulmonary diagnoses seek palliative care, effective management of cardiorespiratory symptoms is becoming an essential component of palliative medicine. Common cardiorespiratory symptoms experienced by many patients with advanced or terminal illness include dyspnea, respiratory secretions, cough, hemoptysis, chest pain, and symptoms secondary to anemia.

Acute care typically includes resuscitation attempts for terminally ill cardiac patients and ventilator support for pulmonary patients. In both situations, extending life is the primary consideration. In palliative care settings, extending life is not the primary consideration; instead, the goal of treatment is to improve the patient's quality of life as much as possible until a comfortable death occurs.

Dyspnea

Dyspnea is an unpleasant sensation of breathing due to a variety of causes, each of which may require specific treatment modalities. Ten percent of cancer patients and 70 percent of lung cancer patients experience dyspnea during the course of their illness,

with the incidence increasing during the last six weeks of life.

The most common causes of malignancy-associated dyspnea are superior vena cava syndromes, airway obstruction, lymphangitic spread of disease to lungs, pulmonary embolism, pleural effusion, pneumonia, anxiety, and anemia. Common causes of noncancer-related dyspnea include congestive heart failure, pulmonary edema, and chronic obstructive pulmonary disease.

The National Hospice Study recognizes underlying cardiac disease and low performance status as additional risk factors for dyspnea, although they are usually associated with pulmonary involvement.

Treatments for superior vena cava syndrome and airway obstruction include radiation therapy, steroids, and opioids. For patients with a life expectancy greater than four weeks, radiation therapy is the definitive treatment; otherwise, palliative treatment with morphine and steroids is more appropriate. Steroids are used to decrease associated tumor edema. In certain clinical scenarios, stent placement may be useful to relieve airway obstruction or hemoptysis.

Lymphangitic spread is characterized by coughing and dyspnea. Treatment consists of controlling the cough and giving morphine and steroids for treatment of dyspnea.

Pulmonary emboli are usually rapid terminal events. Palliative measures include the administration of morphine and sedation.

Patients near the end of life are seldom candidates for heparinization.

Pleural effusions, whether or not secondary to malignancy, may cause significant dyspnea. Depending on the clinical scenario, palliative treatments may include thoracentesis or pleurodesis.

Pneumonia was referred to as the *old man's friend* before the advent of antibiotics. Symptoms of pneumonia include chest pain, secretions associated with a change in color, and increased temperature. Treatment goals should be discussed with patients and families prior to initiating therapy; the most humane treatment for patients with less than two weeks to live may be comfort care without antibiotics.

Congestive heart failure (CHF) is a common cause of dyspnea in end-stage cardiac patients. Signs and symptoms of CHF include dyspnea on exertion, orthopnea, paroxysmal nocturnal dyspnea, fatigue, tachycardia, palpitations, chest pain, jugular venous distension, ascites, peripheral edema, bilateral moist fine crackles at bases, and expiratory wheezes. Treatment of acute CHF may include a combination of oxygen, benzodiazepines, diuretics, nitrates, or morphine sulfate. After an acute episode is resolved, predisposing factors should be assessed and corrected, if possible. Assess patients for maximization of cardiac medications.

Chronic obstructive pulmonary disease (COPD) is characterized by dyspnea associated with conversation, activities of daily living or at rest, weight loss, and muscle wasting. Cor pulmonale or right heart failure may be secondary to advanced COPD, and is manifested by lower extremity edema and electrocardiogram and echocardiogram changes consistent with cor pulmonale. Signs of limited prognosis associated with end-stage COPD are an FEV_1 of less than 30 percent of the predicted value (post use of bronchodilatators), a decline in FEV_1 greater than 40 ml/yr, a PaO_2 less than 55, a SaO_2 of 88 percent or less on O_2, and a $PaCO_2$ greater than 50. The goal of treatment is to relieve dyspnea

and improve oxygen saturation to 88-90 percent. Usual treatments for COPD include anticholinergics (ipatropium bromide), beta agonists (metaproterenol, albuterol), xanthines (aminophylline, theophylline), steroids, morphine, and oxygen. Beta agonists are particularly useful for treating asthma, which is not usually a component of end-stage COPD.

Oxygen is the usual therapy for dyspnea but there is little objective evidence of its benefit, except in patients with COPD or other hypoxic conditions. In some cases, oxygen may provide considerable psychological benefit to patients and their family members. Withholding oxygen when it provides more psychological than physiological benefit is a controversial issue.

Morphine and other opioids may help relieve dyspnea, regardless of etiology. Respiratory depression does not occur when opiates are individually titrated upward in a stepwise fashion. When morphine is used to control dyspnea, improvements typically occur without changes in respiratory rate or oxygen saturation levels. Using morphine to relieve dyspnea in dying patients is safe and effective, and should be considered the standard of care when treating breathlessness.

Morphine can be administered orally, rectally, subcutaneously, or intravenously. The usual starting dose of morphine is 2.5-5 mg orally or sublingually every four hours. For morphine-naïve patients, morphine is administered as needed to relieve symptoms. Some patients respond well to standard preparations of long-acting morphine. When morphine is administered subcutaneously or intravenously, the usual starting dose is 1-2 mg every 3-4 hours.

Morphine may affect respiratory sensation in six ways: it provides cerebral sedation, reduces anxiety, reduces sensitivity to hypercapnia, improves cardiac function, provides analgesia, and (when inhaled) may act on airway opioid receptors. The exact mechanism by which morphine relieves dyspnea is unknown. Morphine may bind with opioid receptors in the lung, altering the central perception of breathlessness and reducing anxiety. Morphine also diminishes ventilatory response to hypoxia and hypercapnia. The vasodilatory effects of morphine reduce preload and may be as efficacious as other routes of administration in the cardiac patient.

Nebulized morphine to relieve dyspnea in terminally ill patients is widely used despite the lack of double-blind placebo controlled studies proving its efficacy. One of the benefits of using nebulized morphine is its low rate of systemic absorption (approximately 5%), thus avoiding most systemic effects. Formulations and dosages of nebulized morphine vary; the most widely accepted dose is a mix of 5-20 mg of parenteral morphine with 3 cc of normal saline, nebulized every four hours as needed. Opioid-naive patients begin with doses of 2.5-5 mg morphine. Hydromorphone can be substituted for morphine, at approximately 10 percent of the morphine dose. Advantages of using hydromorphone include the availability of preservative-free formulations and avoidance of the additional cost of formulating preservative-free morphine.

When breathlessness is secondary to anxiety, careful assessments are needed to determine contributing causes, for example, medications, pulmonary invasion, and/or death-related concerns. Anxiety typically responds to the judicious use of counseling and benzodiazepines. Benzodiazepines induce global cerebral sedation, reduce dyspnea, and depress ventilatory drive. The sedative effects of benzodiazepines may relieve breathlessness associated with respiratory muscle fatigue, by allowing patients much needed rest. Lorazepam is the benzodiazepine of choice due to its short action and sublingual absorption in low dosage forms.

Steroids are widely used to palliate the symptoms of COPD, airway obstruction, superior vena cava syndrome, pulmonary lymphatic spread of malignancy, and bronchospasm. Rapidly tapered dexamethasone is an effective treatment, as is a prednisone pulse for five to seven days, which may be used without tapering. When bronchospasms or pulmonary fibrosis are contributors to dyspnea, solumedrol can be added to the nebulizer treatment. A steroid inhaler with a spacer can also be used. Tuberculosis and active peptic ulcer disease are contraindications to the use of steroids. Due to potential adverse effects, careful individual monitoring is required whenever steroids are used.

Sedation may be necessary to control refractory severe dyspnea, uncontrolled massive hemoptysis, pulmonary emboli, or acute unresolvable airway obstruction. Effective sedating agents include midazolam 1 mg/hr intravenously or subcutaneously titrated to effect, pentobarbital, thorazine, phenobarbital, pentothal, and propofol. Propofol can be added to a continuous infusion of morphine.

Respiratory Secretions

Increased respiratory secretions (death rattle) may occur during the active stage of dying. Usually, patients are not bothered by the secretions, but staff and family often become increasingly uncomfortable. Suctioning should be avoided; it irritates the airway (and the patient), leading to increased production of secretions. More effective treatments include sublingual or oral hyoscyamine, scopolamine patches, atropine, or glycopyrrolate. A continuous infusion of scopolamine subcutaneously or intravenously may also be effective.

Cough

Studies indicate the prevalence of cough may be as high as 83 percent, making it one of the most common symptoms experienced by terminally ill patients. For treatment of productive cough, consider antibiotics if life expectancy is greater than two weeks and the patient desires treatment. Otherwise, first-line treatment is guiafenesin in liquid or long-acting forms. If cough continues, use guiafenesin with codeine. If cough remains uncontrolled, use nebulized acetylcystein and/or nebulized morphine. For patients with non-productive cough, assess for acetylcholinesterase inhibitors as a contributing cause. The first-line treatment for non-productive cough is guiafenesin with dextromethorphan and/or benzonatate perles. If cough continues, use a preparation containing codeine or hydrocodone. If cough remains problematic, use nebulized morphine. Alternatively, nebulized bupivicaine or lidocaine every four hours may be an effective treatment for refractory cough.

Hemoptysis

Patients with chronic lung disease and pulmonary malignancies commonly experience hemoptysis of varying amounts, from scant to massive. Treating cough may resolve the predisposing factor of hemoptysis. Anecdotal reports about the effectiveness of aminocaproic acid indicate mixed results. Massive hemoptysis is an urgent symptom requiring aggressive comfort measures, including morphine or other opioids parenterally by slow intravenous injection, benzodiazepines such as midazolam or lorazepam for sedation (alternately, pentobarbital rectally may be used for sedation), and covering all signs of blood with dark towels to decrease the patient's and family's fear and anxiety.

Chest Pain

Common causes of chest pain include cardiac ischemia, pneumothorax, pulmonary emboli, thoracic aortic dissection, costochondritis, herpes zoster, esophagitis, and peptic ulcer disease. Cardiac ischemic pain is characterized by a pressing, squeezing, weight-like substernal chest pain that sometimes radiates

to the left arm or jaw. Patients may describe the pain as feeling like a clenched fist. Common associated symptoms are dyspnea, confusion, paresthesias, syncope, anxiety, indigestion, nausea, vomiting and diaphoresis. Treatments include nitrates and oxygen. If pain is not relieved by nitrates, morphine sulfate should be administered and repeated until relief is obtained. Chronic unremitting angina may require a subcutaneous morphine pump.

Pneumothorax occurs in patients with pulmonary carcinoma, COPD, and pulmonary fibrosis. It is characterized by decreased breath sounds over the affected lung. If the patient is not imminently dying, a chest tube may be indicated. Opioids are used to relieve pain and dyspnea and, if necessary, benzodiazepines are initiated to relieve anxiety and/or induce sedation.

Pulmonary embolism should be suspected in patients with acute dyspnea, tachycardia and a history of deep venous thrombosis, previous pulmonary emboli, malignancy, or immobilization. Before instituting anticoagulation therapy, consider its contraindications and the patient's life expectancy and ability to undergo necessary diagnostic tests.

Costochondritis, or Tietze's syndrome, is a common cause of chest pain, and often mimics cardiac ischemic pain. Costochondritis is differentiated by tenderness of the chest wall and pain reproduced by palpating the intercostal areas. Nonsteroidals provide dramatic relief.

Herpes zoster can cause pain often described as itching and burning. Herpes zoster may be accompanied by chills, fever, malaise, and a vesicular eruption along a dermatome. Pain may precede the rash by three to four days. To prevent the sequelae of post-herpetic neuralgia, herpes zoster must be treated within 72 hours with acylovir or famciclovir.

Thoracic aortic dissection is characterized by sudden, severe tearing central in the chest. Palliative measures for terminal pulmonary events such as thoracic aortic dissection include morphine via nebulizer, morphine subcutaneously or intravenously until pain is relieved, lorazepam until anxiety is relieved, and pentobarbital suppositories or midazolam if terminal sedation is appropriate.

Gastrointestinal symptoms such as esophagitis, peptic ulcer disease, and cholecystitis also may present as chest pain (see Module 10). Esophagitis pain may be temporally associated with eating, and patients may be aware of acid regurgitation. Patients with a history of peptic ulcer disease and/or use of steroids or nonsteroidals may experience epigastric tenderness, with lessening of pain after eating. Urgent treatment with sucralfate usually brings relief.

Anemia

In terminally ill patients, anemia is most frequently associated with neoplastic and renal disease. Malignancy-related anemia is usually secondary to bone marrow replacement by tumor, bone marrow failure secondary to radiation and/or chemotherapy, or blood loss from bleeding at the tumor site. Signs and symptoms of anemia include fatigue, dyspnea, and tachycardia. Ambulatory patients who benefited from previous transfusions may warrant repeat transfusions.

The quality of life of ambulatory patients with angina, dyspnea at rest, or syncope related to anemia may be improved with transfusion. Transfusions before special events such as weddings, anniversaries, or graduations can be efficacious. Regardless of hemoglobin levels, active bleeding or asymptomatic anemia are never reasons for transfusing terminally ill patients—during the last phase of life, transfusions administered for asymptomatic anemia do not improve the quality of life. Typically, death secondary to blood loss is painless. Intervening with transfusions is unlikely to be successful and may result in the patient experiencing a more unpleasant death at a later time.

Objectives

Attitudes/Behaviors

1. Describe the philosophy of palliation of cardiorespiratory symptoms.

2. Differentiate between uses of benzodiazepines for anxiety-associated dyspnea and for typical anxiety.

3. Describe appropriate use of transfusion in palliative care.

4. Explain a rationale for withholding transfusion for a terminally ill patient with a hemoglobin of six.

5. Explain appropriate and inappropriate use of oxygen therapy in terminally ill patients.

6. Defend the use of morphine for relief of cardiopulmonary symptoms.

7. Defend the use of sedation and analgesics during massive hemoptysis.

8. Develop a treatment plan for a patient with congestive heart failure in a palliative care unit, and compare it with a treatment plan for a similar patient in a coronary care unit.

9. Explain why suctioning is not the treatment of choice for relieving increased respiratory secretions.

10. Justify ordering radiation therapy for a terminally ill patient with superior vena cava syndrome.

11. Describe appropriate treatment for a patient with brittle end-stage congestive heart failure who fails to maintain dietary sodium restrictions.

Knowledge

1. Describe two useful steroid regimes for dyspnea.

2. Describe several causes of dyspnea associated with malignancy.

3. Identify six effects of morphine on respiratory sensation.

4. List three causes of malignancy-related anemia.

5. Describe the treatment of massive hemoptysis.

6. Describe six causes of non-cardiac chest pain.

7. Describe the importance of early treatment of herpes zoster.

8. Describe two treatments for increased respiratory secretions.

9. List three medications used for sedation.

10. Describe indications for the use of nebulized opiates.

Skills

1. Demonstrate appropriate management of a terminally ill patient with a suspected pulmonary embolism.

2. Demonstrate effective communication skills when discussing appropriate treatments for respiratory secretions with family members.

3. Demonstrate an effective step-wise approach for treating nonproductive cough.

4. Utilize effective morphine dosing for a morphine-naïve patient.

5. Effectively manage dyspnea in patients with end-stage COPD.

6. Effectively manage secretions in patients with terminal lung cancer.

7. Effectively manage dyspnea and chest pain in patients with end-stage cardiomyopathy.

8. Utilize intravenous and nebulized morphine when treating dyspnea.

9. Determine the cause of chest pain in a terminally ill patient.

References

1. Ahmedz, S. Palliation of respiratory symptoms. In: Doyle D, Hanks GWC, MacDonald N, eds. *Oxford Textbook of Palliative Medicine*. New York: Oxford University Press; 1993:349-75.

2. Anemia. In: *Medical Care of the Dying*, 2nd ed. Victoria, British Columbia: Victoria Hospice Society; 1993:320-322.

3. Bruera E, MacEachern T, et. al. Subcutaneous morphine for dyspnea in cardiac patients. *Ann Inter Med*.1993;119:906-7.

4. Davis CL, Lam W, Butcher M, et. al. Low systemic bioavailability of nebulized morphine: potential therapeutic role for the relief of dyspnea. *Br J Cancer*. 1992;65:12. Supplement 16.

5. Farncombe M, Charter S. Case studies outlining use of nebulized morphine for patients with end-stage chronic lung and cardiac disease. *J Pain Symptom Manage*. 1993;8(4):221-225.

6. Johanson GA. *Physicians Handbook of Symptom Relief in Terminal Care*, 4th ed. Santa Rosa, Calif: Sonoma County Academic Foundation for Excellence in Medicine; 1994.

7. Levy M. Sedation in Palliative Care: A Fine Intentional Line. Presented at the Ninth Annual Assembly of the American Academy of Hospice and Palliative Medicine. June, 1997; Chicago, Ill.

8. Monti M, Castellanni L, Berlusconi A, Cunietti E. Use of red blood cell transfusions in terminally ill cancer patients admitted to a palliative care unit. *J Pain Symptom Manage*. 1996;12(1):18-22.

9. Ottaviani AN. End Stage Pulmonary Disease. Presented at the Hospice Symposium. Change: Creating Opportunity From Chaos, August 19, 1997; Orlando, Fla.

10. Reuben, DB, Mor V. Dyspnea in terminally ill cancer patients. *Chest*. 1986; 89:234-236.

11. Rousseau P. Management of dyspnea in the dying elderly. *Clin Geriatric*. 1997;5(6):42-43.

12. Stegman MB. Improving cardiac care at end of life. Presented at the Hope Hospice and Palliative Care Breakthrough Series: Collaborative on Improving Care At End of Life. 1997; Fort Myers, Fla.

13. Stegman, MB. *Pain and Symptom Control in Palliative Medicine*. Fort Myers, Fla: Hope Hospice and Palliative Care; 1997.

14. Stein W, Min UK. Nebulized morphine for paroxysmal cough and dyspnea in a nursing home resident with metastatic cancer. *Am J Hospice Palliat Care*. 1997;13(2):52-56.

15. Watanabe, S. Grey Nuns Community Health Centre, Pallative Care Program. Palliative Care Tips: Dyspnea. Issue # 4: August 1996: http://www.palliative.org/@_dyspnea.html

MODULE TEN

Evaluation and Management of Gastrointestinal Symptoms

Common Gastrointestinal Symptoms

Gastrointestinal symptoms are prevalent among patients with advanced progressive disease, and contribute to worsening quality of life and increased stress among caregivers. Symptoms generally occur as a result of underlying disease or are secondary to treatment. Common gastrointestinal symptoms include xerostomia, stomatitis, alteration of taste, dyspepsia, dysphagia, nausea and vomiting, constipation, diarrhea, bowel obstruction, ascites, and hiccups (singultus).

Xerostomia

The prevalence of xerostomia, or dry mouth, among terminally ill patients is unknown, although approximately 40 percent of patients admitted to a hospice program complain of dry mouth. Xerostomia commonly results from three conditions: decreased production of saliva (e.g., dehydration, radiotherapy, drugs), damage to the buccal mucosa (e.g., infection, mucositis, tumor infiltration), and excessive evaporation of saliva (e.g., mouth breathing, oxygen use). Xerostomia can cause pain and discomfort, impaired taste, intolerance to dental prostheses, and difficult mastication and swallowing.

Physical examination may reveal findings such as viscous saliva (after radiotherapy), a dry, smooth tongue and mucosa, erythema, evidence of mucositis or candidiasis, and caked food and mucosal debris.

Appropriate treatment of xerostomia depends on the stage and prognosis of the underlying disease and often involves the following: (1) stimulating salivary flow using items such as lemon drops or pineapple chunks, or the drug pilocarpine; (2) using saliva substitutes; (3) providing good oral care and fluoride use; and (4) offering sips of water or using a spray bottle to lubricate the oral cavity.

Stomatitis

The prevalence of stomatitis in patients with advanced disease is unknown. Stomatitis is caused by chemotherapy, radiotherapy, xerostomia, poor oral hygiene, malnutrition, infection (e.g., fungal, viral, bacterial, apthous), and drugs (e.g., corticosteroids, antibiotics, anticholinergics). The main symptom of stomatitis is pain. Physical examination may reveal varying degrees of erythema, excoriation, ulceration, mucosal bleeding, inflammation, infection, or ulceration of the mucosal membranes. Appropriate treatments depend on the underlying cause and may include good oral hygiene, oral anesthetics, antifungals, and pain medication.

Alteration of Taste

Alteration of taste reportedly affects 25 percent to 50 percent of terminally ill patients; it can result in poor intake and digestion, dehydration, and malnutrition. Taste may be reduced (hypogeusia), lost (ageusia), or distorted (dysgeusia), and can involve one or more taste sensations. Alteration of taste is caused by oral pathology (e.g., tumor, glossectomy, palatectomy, stomatitis) cranial nerve dysfunction, metabolic disturbances (e.g., renal failure, diabetes mellitus), radiotherapy, and drugs (e.g., chemotherapy).

Appropriate interventions include treating the underlying cause, providing good oral care, preparing and presenting foods requested by the patient, manipulating the diet (e.g., less red meat, more dairy products, foods at room temperature), avoiding noxious smells, and using appetite stimulants, including alcohol.

Dyspepsia

Dyspepsia is a term used to describe a variety of symptoms, including epigastric fullness, upper abdominal or retrosternal pain, nausea and/or vomiting, "heartburn," and "regurgitation." The most common causes of dyspepsia in terminally ill patients include reflux esophagitis, gastric hypomotility, peptic ulcer disease, squashed stomach syndrome, and aerophagia. Approximately half of patients with non-ulcer dyspepsia have gastric hypomotility with delayed gastric emptying.

A careful history may reveal the underlying cause. For example, symptoms occurring during or immediately after eating suggests esophageal disease, discomfort after eating suggests peptic ulcer disease, and constant pain may indicate malignant infiltration. Physical examination is usually nondiagnostic. In select cases, radiologic or endoscopic evaluation may be necessary to aid diagnosis; however, invasive and uncomfortable procedures should be performed only after consideration of the stage and prognosis of the underlying disease and careful analysis of the likely benefits and burdens of the procedure.

Treatments include measures to relieve symptoms (e.g., elevation of the head of the bed, frequent small meals), withdrawal of offending drugs (e.g., NSAIDs, anticholinergics), and management of the underlying disorder. Frequently, treatment is empiric and includes the use of antacids, mucosal protective agents (e.g., sucralfate), H_2-receptor antagonists, acid pump inhibitors, a prostaglandin analogue (e.g., misoprostol), and prokinetic agents such as metoclopramide or cisapride.

Dysphagia

Among patients with advanced cancer, the incidence of dysphagia varies from 10 percent to 23 percent, with the highest incidence occurring among patients with cancers of the head and neck, esophagus, stomach, and involvement of the mediastinal and pharyngeal lymph nodes. All three phases of swallowing— buccal, pharyngeal, and esophageal—can be affected by disease, tumor effects, surgical interventions, neuromuscular dysfunction, infections, and radiation. Dysphagia during the esophageal phase of swallowing may be caused by reflux, drug-induced dystonia, weakness and general debility, xerostomia, stomatitis, anxiety, lethargy, sedation, and dementia.

A careful medical history may reveal the etiology of dysphagia. For example, obstructive lesions generally cause dysphagia with solids early in the disease process, neurologic dysfunction produces difficulty with both solids and liquids, and odynophagia (pain with swallowing) suggests inflammation or infection, but may also occur with malignant invasion. Physical examination may be normal or reveal oral lesions, neurologic abnormalities, choking, coughing, or nasal regurgitation of food. Depending on the stage and prognosis of the disease, evaluation may also include a chest x-ray, barium swallow, computerized axial tomography of the chest, and endoscopy.

Dysphagia in 60 percent of patients with cancer can be relieved using conservative treatments, such as offering frequent small meals or semi-liquid diets and sitting patients in an upright position while eating. If the etiology of dysphagia can be identified, treatment should be directed at the underlying cause and may include good oral hygiene, antifungals, dexamethasone (for perineural tumor infiltration and peritumor edema of esophageal malignancies), alternative routes of feeding (e.g., gastrostomy tube), radiotherapy, esophageal dilatation or laser therapy, and insertion of an endo-esophageal tube.

Nausea and Vomiting

Nausea and vomiting (NV) occur in 62 percent of patients with advanced cancer. Up to 60 percent of patients receiving opioid therapy experience NV, particularly during the initiation of therapy. Vomiting is controlled by the vomiting center, which is located in the lateral reticular formation of the medulla. The vomiting center receives input from five sources, each of which is stimulated by specific events:

- Chemoreceptor trigger zone (CTZ): Uremia, chemotherapeutic agents, radiation, opioids, and blood-borne toxins
- Pharynx and gastrointestinal tract: Gastroparesis, extrinsic compressions of the stomach, intestinal obstruction, drugs, radiation, and infection and inflammation
- Cerebral cortex: Anxiety, fear, adverse responses to sounds, sights, and smells
- Vestibular system: Tumors and metastases to base of skull, motion, and dehydration
- Intracranial pressure receptors: Increased intracranial pressure

Many factors contribute to NV in patients with advanced disease. Unless the disease is far advanced and death is imminent, attempts should be made to identify underlying causes and contributing factors.

A concise history and physical examination, including oral, abdominorectal, and neurologic assessments, coupled with minimal laboratory studies such as serum creatinine, urea nitrogen, electrolytes, calcium, and appropriate drug levels, will frequently identify the cause(s) of NV. Nevertheless, empiric therapy is often necessary. Six categories of antiemetics are used to treat NV: antihistamines, anticholinergics, corticosteroids, benzodiazepines, dopamine antagonists, and serotonin antagonists. Non-pharmacologic interventions are also useful, including dietary manipulation (e.g., food served at room temperature, avoiding foods with a strong odor), relaxation techniques, distractions, and fresh air.

Constipation

Constipation, defined as the passage of hard stool, less than the usual number of bowel movements, or infrequent stools (less than every three days), occurs in 40 percent to 90 percent of terminally ill patients. More than 80 percent of hospice patients require laxatives to maintain bowel movements. In the terminally ill population, constipation often is multifactorial and may include:

- Opioid use, which is one of the most common precipitants, and other medications, such as anticholinergics and NSAIDs
- Tumor effects, e.g., obstruction, cauda equina syndrome and metabolic complications, e.g., hypercalcemia
- Concurrent illnesses, debilitation with inactivity, dehydration, weakness, and confusion.

In addition to complaints of infrequent bowel movements or hard stool, patients may complain of rectal pain, abdominal fullness, colic, anorexia, nausea and vomiting, and urinary retention. Occasionally, a severely constipated patient may complain of diarrhea, which usually consists of excess mucus caused by fecal impaction or watery stool which has gone around the impaction.

Physical examination should focus on the abdominal and rectal areas, with special attention to abdominal tenderness, fecal masses, hard impacted stools, and rectal pathology. Further investigation is rarely necessary, although a plain radiograph of the abdomen may confirm clinical suspicions of constipation.

Treatments include laxative therapy, generally with a stool softener and contact cathartic such as senna, substituting less constipating drugs where possible, correcting contributing metabolic abnormalities, encouraging ambulation and adequate fluid intake, providing comfort and privacy for stool evacuation, and if feasible, increasing dietary fiber. Anorexic patients tend to prefer low-fiber foods and are unable to cope with high-fiber diets. If fecal impaction is present, manual disimpaction may be necessary but if soft stool is present, a suppository or enema should be prescribed to empty the rectal vault.

Diarrhea

Diarrhea, defined as more than three or four loose stools a day, occurs in 10 percent of hospice patients and contributes to dehydration, electrolyte disturbances, malnutrition, and pressure ulcer formation. Laxative use is the most common cause of diarrhea in cancer patients. Other causes include bowel obstruction, fecal impaction, malabsorption, infectious agents, drugs (e.g., antibiotics, antacids, iron), AIDS (e.g., bacterial, protozoal, viral pathogens), radiotherapy, prior gastrointestinal surgery, hemorrhage, hormonal-producing tumors, and concurrent medical illnesses.

Physical examination should concentrate on the abdominal and rectal areas, and may be supplemented by abdominal radiography, stool culture and Gram stain, and studies for *Clostridium difficile* if there is a history of prior antibiotic use.

Treatment is directed at underlying causes and general supportive measures, including discontinuing laxatives, maintaining hydration (if possible), protecting the perianal area with products such as topical zinc or cortisone preparations, and using antidiarrheal agents.

Bowel Obstruction

Malignant bowel obstruction, also covered in Module 7, occurs in 3 percent of all terminally ill cancer patients, with obstruction particularly common in ovarian (5.5% to 42%) and colorectal (10% to 28.4%) malignancies. Physical examination often reveals varying degrees of abdominal distention with normal-to-hyperactive bowel sounds, although in the latter stages of obstruction, bowel sounds may be absent. Rectal examination may be normal or reveal hard, impacted stool. In ambiguous cases, plain abdominal radiographs, barium studies, and endoscopy may be diagnostically useful, particularly in patients with a prognosis of prolonged survival.

Appropriate treatment of malignant bowel obstruction depends on life expectancy and may involve nasogastric intubation, surgery, and symptomatic therapy (i.e., opioid analgesics, anticholinergics, antiemetics, corticosteroids, octreotide). With available pharmacologic treatments, the use of nasogastric tubes may be avoided.

Ascites

Ascites occurs in 15 percent to 50 percent of patients with cancer and 6 percent of patients entering a hospice program. Malignant peritoneal infiltration accounts for more than 50 percent of cases, with tumor invasion of liver parenchyma occurring in 15 percent. Ascites may also be secondary to nonmalignant ailments such as cardiac or hepatic disease. A careful history often reveals complaints of increasing abdominal girth, weight gain, pedal and genital edema, indigestion, bloating, early satiety, NV, dyspnea, and orthopnea.

Physical examination may be normal with mild ascites, or reveal bulging flanks with larger amounts of fluid. Occasionally, when such work-ups are necessary and appropriate, ultrasound, or computed axial tomographs of the liver are needed to detect small volumes of fluid. Diagnostic paracentesis may also be necessary to ascertain the nature of the ascites (malignant vs. nonmalignant). Treatment involves management of the underlying disorder, salt and water restriction, diuretics such as spironolactone and furosemide in mild ascites, paracentesis for tense ascites, and possibly, a peritoneovenous shunt. Radiation therapy may also be considered if a demonstrable mass obstructs lymphatic drainage in the mediastinum or retroperitoneum.

Hiccups

Hiccups, or singultus, is a common phenomenon in patients with advanced disease. More than 100 causes of hiccups exist but they can be categorized as follows: (1) disorders affecting the peripheral branches of the phrenic and vagal nerves, (2) central nervous system disorders, (3) metabolic and drug-induced etiologies, (4) infectious disorders, (5) psychogenic disturbances, and (6) idiopathic causes. In dying patients, gastric distention is probably the most common cause of hiccups.

Physical examination and laboratory evaluations usually are nondiagnostic for determining etiology of hiccups; consequently, treatment is frequently empiric. Numerous non-pharmacologic and pharmacologic maneuvers can attenuate hiccups. Since most patients have already tried non-pharmacologic home remedies, pharmacologic agents such as the following are usually prescribed: neuroleptics, prokinetic agents, anticonvulsants, and baclofen.

Objectives

Attitudes/Behaviors

1. Explain the effects of gastrointestinal symptoms on the quality of life of patients and family members.

2. Describe the importance of a non-curative approach to *most* gastrointestinal symptoms.

3. Explain how physical gastrointestinal symptoms affect social, psychological, and spiritual suffering.

4. Discuss why treatment for the same problem may differ depending on a patient's life expectancy.

5. Explain the importance of noninvasive treatment of bowel obstruction in patients close to the end of life.

6. Describe the importance of developing a bowel regimen/program for patients on opiates.

Knowledge

1. Identify causes of each of the following symptom: xerostomia, stomatitis, dyspepsia, dysphagia, constipation, diarrhea, NV, bowel obstruction, hiccup.

2. Discuss the pathophysiology of each gastrointestinal symptom listed above.

3. Describe the physical findings (if applicable) for each symptom listed above.

4. Identify appropriate laboratory and radiographic studies useful for assessing the gastrointestinal symptoms listed above.

5. List pharmacologic and non-pharmacologic treatments for each gastrointestinal symptom listed above.

6. List various causes of ascites in the terminally ill patient.

7. Describe treatment approaches for patients with ascites.

8. Describe causes of diarrhea in a patient with fecal impaction.

Skills

1. Demonstrate the ability to complete a medical history and physical examination relating to the gastrointestinal system.

2. Demonstrate the ability to appropriately utilize laboratory and radiographic studies to assist in the treatment of gastrointestinal symptoms.

3. Exhibit the ability to control gastrointestinal symptoms by choosing appropriate treatment.

4. Demonstrate the ability to communicate with terminally ill patients regarding gastrointestinal symptoms and their treatment.

5. Demonstrate the ability to collaborate with medical, nursing, and allied health professionals, and to share information about gastrointestinal symptoms, including but not limited to diagnosis and treatment.

6. Initiate standard treatment for bowel obstruction for patients close to the end of life.

7. Manage the iatrogenic causes of NV in patients with advanced disease.

8. Treat a patient with fecal impaction

References

1. Allan SG. Emesis in the patient with advanced cancer. *Palliat Med*. 1988;2:89-100.
2. Ashby MA, Game PA, Devitt P, et al. Percutaneous gastrostomy as a venting procedure in palliative care. *Palliat Med*. 1991;5:147-150.
3. Baines M. Nausea and vomiting in the patient with advanced cancer. *J Pain Symptom Manage*. 1988;3:81-85.
4. Baines M, Oliver DJ, Catre RL. Medical management of intestinal obstruction in patients with advanced malignant disease—a clinical and pathological study. *Lancet*. 1985;2:990-993.
5. Billings JA. Anorexia. *J Palliat Care*. 1994;10(1):51-53.

6. Bhandari R, Burakoff R. A pharmacological approach to secretory diarrhea. *Gastroenterologist*. 1995;3:67-74.
7. Bhattacharya I. Evaluation and management of dyspepsia. *Hosp Pract*. 1992;27(10A):3-96,100-101.
8. Bruera E. Current pharmacological management of anorexia in cancer patients. *Oncology*. 1992;6:125-130.
9. Bruera E. Clinical management of cachexia and anorexia in patients with advanced cancer. *Oncology*. 1992;49 (Suppl 2):35-42.
10. Bruera E, MacDonald RN. Nutrition in cancer patients: an update and review of our experience. *J Pain Symptom Manage*. 1988;3:133-140.
11. Carl W. Oral complications of local and systemic cancer treatment. *Curr Opin Oncol*. 1995;7:320-324.
12. DeConno F, Ripamonti C, Sbanatto A, Ventafridda V. Oral complications in patients with advanced cancer. *J Palliat Care*. 1989; 5:7-15.
13. Dose AM. The symptom experience of mucositis, stomatitis, and xerostomia. *Semin Oncol Nurs*. 1995;11:248-255.
14. Doyle D, Hanks GWC, MacDonald N, eds. *Oxford Textbook of Palliative Medicine*. 2nd ed. New York: Oxford University Press; 1997.
15. Enck RE. *The Medical Care of Terminally Ill Patients*. Baltimore: Johns Hopkins Press, 1994.
16. Fainsinger RL, Spachynski K, Hanson J, et. al. Symptom control in terminally ill patients with malignant bowel obstruction (MBO). *J Pain Symptom Manage*. 1994;9:12-18.
17. Hogan CM. Advances in the management of nausea and vomiting. *Nurs Clin North Am*. 1990;25(2):475-497.
18. Howard RS. Persistent hiccups. *BMJ*. 1992;305:1237-1238.
19. Jobbins J, Bagg J, Finlay AG, et al. Oral and dental disease in terminally ill cancer patients. *B MJ*. 1992;304:1612.
20. Krishnasamy M. Oral problems in advanced cancer. *Eur J Cancer Care*. 1995;4:73-177.
21. Levy MH, Catalano RB. Control of common physical symptoms other than pain in patients with terminal disease. *Semin Oncol*. 1985;12:411-430.
22. Lichter I. Nausea and vomiting in patients with cancer. *Hematol Oncol Clin North Am*. 1996;10(1):207-220.
23. Lichter I. Which antiemetic? *J Palliat Care*. 1993;9:42-50.
24. Mercadante S. Diarrhea in terminally ill patients: pathophysiology and treatment. *J Pain Symptom Manage*. 1995; 10:298-309.
25. Moriarty KJ, Irving MH. Constipation. *BMJ*. 1992:304:1237-1240.
26. Nelson KA, Walsh D, Sheehan FA. The cancer anorexia-cachexia syndrome. *J Clin Oncol*. 1994;12: 213-255.
27. Parsons SL, Watson SA, Steele RJ. Malignant ascites. *Br J Surg*. 1996;83:6-14.
28. Poland JM. Stomatitis and specific oral infections of the oncologic patient. *Am J Hospice Care*. 1987; 4:30-32.
29. Portenoy RK. Constipation in the cancer patient: causes and management. *Med Clin North Am*. 1987;71:303-311.
30. Regnard C. Managing dysphagia in advanced cancer—a flow diagram. *Palliat Med*. 1990;4:215.
31. Regnard C. The treatment of bowel obstruction in advanced cancer: an algorithm. *Palliat Med*. 1988;2:131-133.
32. Regnard C, Fitton S. Mouth care: a flow diagram. *Palliat Med*. 1989;3:67-69.
33. Regnard C. Constipation: an algorithm. *Palliat Med*. 1988;2:34-35.
34. Regnard C, Cormisky M. Nausea and vomiting in advanced cancer. *Palliat Med*. 1992;6:146-151.
35. Riley J, Fallon MT. Octreotide in terminal malignant obstruction of the gastrointestinal tract. *Eur J Palliat Care*. 1994;1(1):23-25.
36. Ripamonti C. Management of bowel obstruction in advanced cancer patients. *J Pain Symptom Manage*. 1994;9:193-200
37. Robustelli Della Cunna G, Pelligrini A, Piazzi M. Effect of methylprednisolone sodium succinate on quality of life in pre-terminal cancer patients: a placebo controlled multicenter study. *Eur J Cancer Clin Oncol*. 1989;25:1817-1821.
38. Rousseau PC. Antiemetic therapy in adults with terminal disease: a brief review. *Am J Hospice Palliat Care*. 1995;12:13-18.
39. Rousseau PC. Hiccups in terminal disease. *Am J Hospice Palliat Care*. 1994;11(6):7-10.

---

40. Rousseau PC. Hospice and palliative care. *Dis Mon*. 1995;41(12):769-844.
41. Rousseau PC. Nonpain symptom management in terminal care. *Clin Geriatr Med*. 1996;12(2):313-327.
42. Runyon BA. Care of patients with ascites. *N Engl J Med*. 1994; 330: 337-342.
43. Sharma S, Walsh D. Management of symptomatic malignant ascites with diuretics. Two case reports and a review of the literature. *J Pain Symptom Manage*. 1995; 10:237-242.
44. Siuta M, Sanyal AJ, Schubert ML. Tips for the treatment of refractory ascites. *Gastroenterology*. 1996; 110:956-958.
45. Snyder JD. Evaluation and treatment of diarrhea. *Semin Gastrointest Dis*. 1994;5:47-52.
46. Sykes NP. A clinical comparison of laxatives in a hospice. *Palliat Med*. 1991;5:307-314.
47. Sykes NP. Current approaches to the management of constipation. *Cancer Surv*. 1994;21:137-146.
48. Talley NJ. Modern management of dyspepsia. *Aust Fam Physician*. 1996; 5:47-52.
49. Tchekmedyian NS, Kickman M, Heber D. Treatment of anorexia and weight loss with megestrol acetate in patients with cancer or acquired immunodeficiency syndrome. *Sem Oncol*. 1991;18(1)(suppl 2)(1):35-42.
50. Toomey D, Redmond P, Bouchier-Hayes D. Mechanisms mediating cancer cachexia. *Cancer*. 1995;76:2418-2426.
51. Twycross RG, Lack SA. *Control of Alimentary Symptoms in Far Advanced Cancer*. Edinburgh: Churchill Livingstone; 1986.
52. Watanabe S, Bruera E. Anorexia and cachexia, asthenia, and lethargy. *Hematol Oncol Clin North Am*. 1996;10(1):189-206.
53. Wright PS, Thomas SL. Constipation and diarrhea: the neglected symptoms. *Semin Oncol Nurs*. 1995;11:289-297.

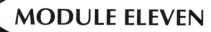

Evaluation and Management of Genitourinary Symptoms

Common Genitourinary Symptoms

In patients with advanced progressive disease, distressing genitourinary symptoms are usually associated with cancer or end-stage renal disease. However, end-stage heart, lung, and neurologic disease may result in significant genitourinary complications requiring aggressive palliative symptom management. This module focuses on palliative treatment of the following symptoms: genitourinary pain, painful micturition, hematuria, urinary incontinence, and obstructive uropathy. Because many profoundly ill patients require urinary tract catheterization for varying lengths of time, indications for indwelling catheters and catheter care are addressed briefly.

Typically, death resulting from end-stage renal disease is accompanied by fewer symptoms than death from other organ system failure. Most patients dying of renal disease become increasingly lethargic and comatose prior to death. To prevent complications of fluid overload, fluids should be administered cautiously to patients with advanced kidney disease and minimal urinary output. Dialysis is rarely indicated or tolerated near the end of life.

Genitourinary Pain

Some genitourinary pain syndromes have unique presentations and are easily diagnosed at the bedside. Others are more difficult to diagnose, particularly when patients are obtunded or non-communicative. In such cases, pain may be indicated by new onset agitation, confusion, or delirium. Usually, genitourinary pain is visceral instead of somatic or neuropathic, but mixed pain can occur and often responds to opiates (see Modules 5 and 6). Paradoxically, use of opioids may create a new problem—urinary retention.

- Renal colic varies from intermittent aching flank pain to the *worst pain* ever experienced. Because renal colic begins when nociceptors in the renal capsule are activated by acute distention, by products of inflammation, or by mechanical distortion, pain may be experienced as a squeezing sensation. Pain often radiates to the ipsilateral inguinal and thigh regions because somatic fibers from those areas enter the spinal cord at the same level as renal afferents. Renal afferents also pass through the vagus nerve and celiac plexus, which explains the nausea, vomiting, and decreased intestinal peristalsis associated with renal colic.
- Pyelonephritis pain tends to be steady, boring, and localized to the flank, with significant costovertebral tenderness. Fever, chills, nausea, vomiting, and dysuria are also associated with pyelonephritis.
- Ureteral pain depends on the location of the obstruction. Typically, upper ureteral pain is abrupt in onset due to obstruction caused

by stones, blood clots, tumor, or necrosed papilla. Lower ureteral pain may be associated with bladder urgency and urinary frequency, and often is experienced in the suprapubic region or the urinary meatus.

During the course of certain malignant diseases with pelvic involvement, gradual asymptomatic obstruction of the lower ureter occurs. Until symptoms of uremia emerge, the only sign of the obstructing process may be decreased urinary output.

- Bladder pain usually occurs in the suprapubic region but may be experienced as unexplained lower back pain, especially among women. Dyes such as phenazopyridine or methylene blue may prove effective as mucosal analgesics.
- Acute prostatitis presents as pain in the lower back and perineum, usually with associated fever, chills, and voiding symptoms. Terminally ill males requiring long-term indwelling catheters are at increased risk for this complication; however, catheters may also eliminate symptoms of dysuria, frequency, and urgency.
- Pain in the scrotal area usually is referred pain from the ureter, trigone, or bladder neck regions. With referred pain, there is no testicular tenderness on physical exam.

Painful Micturition

Painful voiding or dysuria usually is associated with frequent urination, a sense of incomplete bladder emptying, urgency, dribbling, or nocturia. Often, pain is burning in quality and begins with the onset of urination, subsiding at the termination of voiding. Pain occurring at the end of voiding may indicate prostate involvement. In palliative care settings, the most frequent cause of dysuria is urinary infection; however, painful micturition also may result from a stone in the lower

ureter or irritation of the bladder's trigone area. Characteristically, the burning sensation is appreciated at the meatus.

Cervical or ovarian cancers or invading tumors from other contiguous organs also may produce dysuria. Other causes of pain include complications of radiation therapy to the pelvis, cancer chemotherapy, bladder stone, diverticulitis, chronic interstitial cystitis, and chronic prostatitis.

Because terminally ill patients with dysuria frequently are too weak to undergo extensive studies, treatment may be empiric based on the most likely cause of pain. Many patients have chronic indwelling catheters, thus urinary tract infections should be suspected. The incidence of urinary tract infection is related to the duration of catheterization; acquired bacteriuria occurs at a rate of 5 percent per day. Usually, urinalysis with culture can be obtained easily and patients are treated empirically with antibiotics such as trimethoprim-sulfa or amoxicillin, until the culture returns.

Bladder spasms are a variant of dysuria. Patients usually describe the spasms as intermittent episodes of excruciating pain in the suprapubic area, often associated with leakage of urine around an indwelling catheter. Causes of spasm include a build-up of encrustations on the catheter tip or the inflated catheter balloon. Partially deflating the balloon or changing the catheter may help. A urinary analgesic such as phenazopyridine may be all that is necessary to keep the patient comfortable. If pain continues, drugs with anticholinergic action such as oxybutinin hydrochloride, propantheline bromide or belladonna/opium suppositories may be helpful. On occasion, instillation of local anesthetics into the bladder may be needed.

Hematuria

Passing unexpected gross blood, even when asymptomatic, is a frightening experience for most patients. Patients may interpret gross hematuria as the beginning of the terminal event or as a sign of sudden acceleration of their disease. Depending on the clinical scenario, evaluation of gross hematuria may be required. Microscopic hematuria rarely produces as much anxiety. Usually, it can be predicted and does not require extensive evaluation. In the terminally ill population, common causes of gross and/or microscopic hematuria include the following:

- Kidney: cystic disease, benign or malignant neoplasm, stones, renal infarction, glomerulonephritis, pyelonephritis, thrombocytopenia, anticoagulant conditions, or radiation injury
- Ureter: stones, neoplasm, stricture
- Bladder: neoplasm, infection, medications, catheter-induced, stones, varix
- Prostate: neoplasm, engorged vein, infection
- Pseudohematuria: medications, foods, hemoglobinuria, myoglobinuria, bilirubinuria

Important points to consider when evaluating hematuria include:

- Onset of hematuria at initiation of micturition, with clearing toward the end, implies urethral source;
- Hematuria at the end of voiding suggests prostate or bladder source;
- Continuous bleeding implies bladder or higher source;
- Fever with distressing symptoms such as urgency, dysuria, and frequency suggests lower tract infection;
- Fever with flank or abdominal pain implies upper urinary tract infection. Thorough physical examination is required, including rectal and genital exam in men and rectovaginal exam in women.

Depending on the stage of illness, further evaluation of gross hematuria using intravenous pyelography, retrograde pyelography, ultrasound, or CT scan may be necessary. If the diagnosis remains elusive after examining the upper and lower urinary tracts, cystoscopy and other invasive testing may be indicated.

When determining appropriate therapeutic options for hematuria, consideration of invasive investigations to determine etiology should be tempered by consideration of the patient's wishes, condition, prognosis, and the goals of treatment. When possible, palliative treatments should address the underlying diagnosis, but supportive transfusions may be the most appropriate therapy. Recently, fibrinolytic inhibitors such as aminocaproic acid and tranexamic acid have proven effective at controlling cancer-associated bleeding when used systemically or topically instilled in the bladder.

Voiding and Urinary Incontinence

Urinary continence requires functioning higher brain centers, an intact bladder wall, an involuntary internal sphincter at the bladder neck, and a voluntary external sphincter, which is located primarily in the middle third of the female urethra and the distal prostatic urethra of the male. When the bladder wall is extended, stretch receptors of the parasympathetic nerves fire, causing contraction of the detrusor muscle unless inhibited by higher brain centers. At the same time, sympathetic tone at the bladder neck decreases, allowing relaxation and opening of the internal sphincter. Urine flows to the external sphincter, at which time higher brain centers maintain retention or permit expulsion.

Urinary incontinence is the involuntary loss of urine sufficient to cause a social or health problem. The prevalence of urinary incontinence in the terminally ill is unknown. One prospective study of 61 terminally ill cancer patients revealed that 75 percent of patients required an indwelling catheter at some time prior to death.

Common causes of acute urinary incontinence include urinary tract infection, fecal impaction, medication, vaginal prolapse, and mental status changes. Medications affecting continence include the following: diuretics, anticholinergics, antidepressants, antipsychotics, sedative/hypnotics, narcotics, alpha-adrenergic blockers, alpha-adrenergic agonists, beta-adrenergic agonists, and calcium channel blockers.

Chronic urinary incontinence is categorized into four types, which may overlap: stress, urge, overflow, and functional. In hospice/palliative care settings, formal urodynamic testing is problematic and impractical; in most instances, management requires a chronic indwelling catheter. Stress incontinence results from weak pelvic floor musculature or urethral sphincter and usually occurs with increased intraabdominal pressure, for example, coughing and sneezing. Urge incontinence typically is secondary to detrusor hyperactivity due to bladder or urethral inflammation, central nervous system disease, or poor bladder compliance. Anticholinergic medications provide effective treatment for urge incontinence. Overflow incontinence usually occurs with neuropathies, spinal cord tumors, or anatomic obstructions, for example, enlarged prostate, tumor, stricture, cystocele, or impaction. Functional incontinence results from an inability to toilet secondary to impaired cognition or physical functioning, psychological unwillingness, and environmental barriers.

Treatments for various types of urinary incontinence include surgical procedures, pharmacologic therapy, and non-pharmacologic measures such as exercise. As the dying process continues, most terminally ill patients ultimately require either intermittent or chronic catheterization. Prompted voiding or external collection devices may be appropriate for some patients. Staff must be skilled in monitoring urinary output in relation to fluid intake and recognizing the early signs and symptoms of urinary retention, such as restlessness and unexplained new-onset agitation.

Urethral Catheterization

The main indications for indwelling catheterization are (1) bladder outlet obstruction not appropriate for surgical intervention, (2) skin breakdown caused or aggravated by incontinence, (3) neurogenic bladder dysfunction, (4) a need to measure urinary output, (5) increasing weakness as death approaches. Urinary catheter care includes sterile technique, maintenance of a system of closed drainage, and daily perineal care. Due to the presence of asymptomatic bacteriuria in patients with indwelling catheters, specimens for urinalysis or culture should be obtained only from newly inserted or changed catheters.

Obstructive Uropathy

Significant decreases in urinary output, especially with no change in fluid intake, may result in alarmed concern among patients and caregivers. In other cases, it goes unnoticed, which sets the stage for lethal complications.

Three general mechanisms of obstruction are (1) mechanical obstruction of the lumen of the urinary tract from stone, tumor, clot, tissues or crystals; (2) anatomic abnormalities of the ureter, bladder, or urethra such as strictures, or functional abnormalities associated with the use of drugs such as anticholinergics and alpha adrenergic agonists; and (3) compression from masses (most commonly associated with cervical cancer in women and prostatic cancer in men) or processes extrinsic to the urinary tract, such as retroperitoneal fibrosis.

The clinical manifestations of obstruction can be subtle and variable. Urgency, incontinence, nocturia, hesitancy, and unexplained restlessness may indicate pathology of the lower tract, that is, the bladder or distal structures. When obstruction involves the upper tract, such symptoms are not present. Instead, renal pain may be a presenting feature, depending on the rate of obstruction of the upper tract. A slowly dilating pelvis can accommodate large volumes of urine painlessly. Therefore, intermittent flank pain due to acute distension caused by intake of large volumes of fluid should suggest the presence of obstruction. Fever, flank pain, and dysuria suggest infection, which occurs in 8 to 15 percent of non-instrumented patients with obstruction.

Renal failure and the emergence of symptomatic uremic syndromes may be associated with hyperkalemia, acidosis, hypocalcemia, hyperphosphatemia, anemia, impaired immunity, anorexia, nausea, vomiting, mental status changes, and itching. Unilateral obstruction will not produce renal failure if the opposite kidney is functional. Acute oliguric renal failure may result from multiple myeloma and precipitation of Bence-Jones proteins in the tubules, or uric acid crystals that form when patients with myeloproliferative disorders are treated with chemotherapy.

Evaluation for suspected obstruction begins with a thorough history focusing on drug exposure, diagnosis, and knowledge of the disease's likely course and complications. For example, a sudden decrease in urinary output in a female with ovarian cancer or other pelvic malignancy indicates the likelihood of mechanical obstruction. Decreased urine production in an elderly male with lung cancer is more likely to result from medications used to manage other symptoms. Physical examination should focus on the rectum and external genitalia in males and the rectovaginal area in females.

A diagnosis of obstruction is confirmed when the obstruction is relieved by catheterization. Diagnosis may depend on the demonstration of a dilated urinary collecting system. The latter can usually be achieved with noninvasive procedures such as sonography. The goals of therapy for obstructive uropathy depend on the underlying terminal process, the patient's prognosis, the patient's quality of life, and the patient's and/or caregiver's wishes. The benefits and burdens of aggressively pursing a definitive diagnosis and treating the condition must be evaluated from the patient's point of view. Palliative treatment to relieve an obstruction may include an indwelling Foley catheter, a suprapubic catheter, or stent placement if needed.

Objectives

Attitudes/Behaviors

1. Describe the goals of evaluating and treating an obstruction in a terminally ill patient.

2. Justify the use of an indwelling catheter in a terminally ill patient.

3. Explain the evaluation of urinary incontinence in terminally ill patients.

4. Explain the approach to the workup of the terminally ill patient with hematuria.

5. Provide guidance as patients with end-stage renal disease and their family members make decisions regarding the withholding or discontinuing of dialysis.

6. Justify the use of minimal fluids for patients with end-stage renal disease.

Knowledge

1. Differentiate the likely origins of genitourinary pain.

2. Describe differences in kidney, ureteral, and bladder pain.

3. Discuss the presentation of prostate pain.

4. Explain the normal voiding mechanism.

5. Define four major types of chronic urinary incontinence and appropriate treatment for each type.

6. Describe the major causes of acute urinary incontinence.

7. Describe indications for urinary catheterization in terminally ill patients.

8. Identify causes of dysuria in the terminally ill.

9. Discuss the differential diagnosis of gross hematuria.

10. Explain indications for non-invasive evaluation of hematuria.

11. Describe three mechanisms that produce genitourinary tract obstruction.

12. List types of medications that may affect a patient's continence.

13. Discuss the incidence of catheter-related bladder spasm and its treatment.

14. Describe the phenomenon of pseudohematuria.

Skills

1. Treat patients with acute and chronic urinary incontinence.

2. Treat a patient with clinical symptoms of uremia.

3. Evaluate and treat a terminally ill patient with dysuria.

4. Evaluate and treat a terminally ill patient with bladder spasm.

5. Evaluate and treat a terminally ill patient with obstructive uropathy.

6. Manage patients with end-stage renal disease who refuse or discontinue dialysis.

References

1. AHCPR Urinary Incontinence Guidelines Panel. *Urinary Incontinence in Adults: Clinical Practice Guidelines*. AHCPR Pub. No. 92-0038. Rockville MD. Agency for Health Care Policy and Research, Public Health Service, U.S. Department of Health and Human Services. March, 1992.
2. Dean A, Tuffin P: Fibrinolytic inhibitors for cancer-associated bleeding problems. *J Pain Symptom Manage*. 1997;13(1):20-24.
3. Degowin EL, Degowin RL: Hematuria. In: *Bedside Diagnostic Examination*, 3rd ed. New York:Macmillan Publishing Co; 1976:574-576.
4. Elhilali MM, Winfield HN. Genitourinary pain. In: Wall PD, Melzack R, eds. *Textbook of Pain*, 2nd ed, London: Churchill Livingstone; 1989:500-507.
5. Enck RE. The management of urinary incontinence. *Am J Hospice Care*. 1989;6(6):9-10.

6. Fainsinger RL, MacEachern T, et.al. The use of urinary catheters in terminally ill cancer patients. *J Pain Symptom Manage.* 1992;7(6):333-338.

7. Mackinnon KJ, Norman RW: Genitourinary disorders in palliative medicine. In: Doyle D, Hanks GWC, MacDonald N, eds. *Oxford Textbook of Palliative Medicine.* New York: Oxford University Press; 1993:415-421.

8. Ouslander JG: Urinary incontinence. In: Hazzard WR, Andres R, et. al., eds. *Principles of Geriatric Medicine and Gerontology,* 2nd ed. New York: McGraw-Hill Inc; 1990:1123-1142.

9. Rector, Jr. FC. Obstructive uropathy. In: Wyngaarden JB, Smith, Jr. LH, eds. *Cecil Textbook of Medicine,* 18th ed. Philadelphia, Pa: W.B. Saunders Co.; 1988:614-616.

10. Woods DR, Bender BS: Long-term urinary tract catheterization. *Med Clin North Am.* 1989; 73(6):1441-1444.

Evaluation and Management of Neuropsychiatric Symptoms

Neuropsychiatric Symptoms

The neuropsychiatric symptoms encountered in advanced progressive disease are among the most challenging symptoms to manage, due in part to their frequent relationship with coexisting medical conditions. When a patient's decision-making capacity is compromised, management can be particularly challenging.

Nearly half of the patients with cancer experience sustained neuropsychiatric conditions such as anxiety, depression, and disorders of cognitive function. Critical questions to consider are: (1) When does sadness become depression? and (2) When does fear about the future become an anxiety state? Effective management techniques often require the skills of an interdisciplinary team of healthcare professionals.

Emotional Responses to Illness

A person's response to advanced illness is variable and depends on a host of coping mechanisms and strategies, such as regression, denial, rationalization, intellectualization, projection, displacement, introjection, repression, and withdrawal. The acquisition of effective coping mechanisms is influenced by personality, parenting, social supports, communication skills, life experience, and time.

Physicians should include a psychosocial history as part of the patient's history and physical. Information about the patient's background, beliefs, understanding of the world, life experiences, philosophy, expectations, and future hopes or plans should be included. To better understand the patient's and family's coping strategies, it is often useful to inquire about previous life stresses and coping strategies that were used in the past. Information about family deaths or illnesses is invaluable.

Depression

The spectrum of responses to illness and life stress ranges from sadness to transient depression (adjustment disorder) to depressive illness. Clinical depression is grossly underrecognized and undertreated in patients with cancer and HIV disease, partly because healthcare providers mistakenly assume depression is an expected component of advanced disease and should not be treated. Patients should be screened for risk factors, including previous history of affective disorders or alcoholism, poor pain control, mutilating surgery, multiple medical illnesses, social isolation, low socioeconomic status, marital problems, and difficulty expressing anger.

Recognizing the clinical symptoms of major depression is critical. Psychological symptoms include depressed mood, irritability, anhedonia, agitation, psychomotor retardation, and feelings of worthlessness, meaninglessness, and hopelessness. Physical symptoms include fatigue, weakness, sleep disturbance, diurnal mood swing, and appetite disturbances. When evaluating depression in terminally ill patients, physicians should rely more on the patient's psychological symptoms; the usual physical symptoms of depression may not be reliable indicators of depression due to their common occurrence in advanced disease, even when depression is not a factor.

Accumulating research indicates that depression is not a universal symptom of terminal illness, nor is it refractory to management. When depressive illness occurs, it causes great suffering for patients and family members, and warrants vigorous treatment. The diagnosis and management of depression require training and a willingness to refer difficult cases to appropriate mental health professionals. Effective treatments include the following: selective serotonin reuptake inhibitors (SSRIs), tricyclic antidepressants, psychostimulants, and supportive psychotherapy.

Anxiety

Considerable overlap occurs in diagnoses of depression and anxiety disorder. Anxiety is part of the normal human experience; however, when it becomes persistent and severe, anxiety is an illness requiring treatment. Anxiety commonly occurs as a result of the following conditions:

- Incomplete or inadequate psychological defense mechanisms
- Overwhelming stress
- Organic causes, particularly pharmacologic
- Underlying medical problems and unrecognized drug effects, such as alcohol or recreational drug use
- Pain and other distressing symptoms, which must be managed effectively

The type of anxiety state and its causes determine the approach to management, which may include the following:

- Benzodiazepines, which often are first-line treatments
- Antidepressants, neuroleptics, antiepileptics, buspirone, and hydroxyzine, which may be helpful in selected cases
- Supportive psychotherapy and relaxation therapy, which can be invaluable

Suicide

Patients in the advanced stages of terminal illness are at increased risk of suicide relative to the general population. Risk factors for suicide include:

- Depression, helplessness, hopelessness
- Pain, fatigue, delirium, disinhibition
- Pre-existing psychopathology, substance or alcohol abuse
- Previous suicide attempts, family history of suicide, social isolation

Expressions of suicidal thoughts or requests for assistance with suicide by patients or family members should be taken seriously. Discussing suicidal thoughts with patients and family members can be therapeutic, and often decreases the risk of suicide, if the underlying contributors to a desire for suicide are addressed. When distressing symptoms are effectively controlled and skilled practitioners provide psychological and spiritual support, requests for suicide often dissipate.

Delirium and Dementia

Mental confusion commonly occurs during terminal illness and can adversely affect the last stages of a patient's life. Instead of offering a time for continued personal growth and development, the active phases of dying may instead become times of anguish and distress for all concerned. When the patient's confusion is inadequately treated, both the patient and family suffer, which may profoundly affect the family's bereavement.

It is critical to distinguish between delirium and dementia. The Folstein Mini-Mental Status Examination is often used to evaluate patients with cognitive impairment.

Delirium

Delirium is characterized by acute onset with global disorientation, including to time, place, and person, usually with a fluctuating state of arousal.

The causes of delirium should be sought and reversed when possible. Reversible causes include the following: dehydration, hypoxemia, infection, changes in environment, medications, metabolic and electrolyte changes (metabolism of some drugs changes during advanced terminal illness), pain, urinary retention, fecal impaction, and drug withdrawal.

General management strategies include the following:

- Providing quiet, well illuminated surroundings and familiar faces
- Providing hearing aids, spectacles, and clues to orientation, such as calendars and clocks
- Moving the patient to a familiar environment, such as home
- Medications, such as neuroleptics and benzodiazepines

Grieving patients and family members may exhibit grief syndromes that mimic delirium or severe psychiatric disturbances. The decision to use sedating drugs often presents an ethical dilemma for families and caregivers, particularly when the patient is no longer capable of making decisions.

Dementia

Dementia is characterized by its slow progression over time, prominent memory loss, and the rare occurrence of fluctuating consciousness in advanced stages.

The most common causes of dementia are Alzheimer's disease and vascular etiologies, such as multi-infarct dementia. Patients in the advanced stages of dementia may be appropriate for hospice and palliative care services. At advanced stages of disease, patients may lose their ability to ambulate, communicate, eat, and control their bodily functions. Patients with dementing illnesses may also develop delirium and depression.

Hallucinations

Hallucinations may be predominately visual or auditory. In some situations, hallucinations that do not disturb the patient require no medical intervention. Sudden onset of disturbing visual hallucinations may be a side effect of medications such as opiate analgesics, or secondary to an underlying disease process. Opioid rotation may be all that is required in certain scenarios. Persistent disturbing hallucinations may be managed with neuroleptic medications.

Seizures

Seizures may be the first manifestation of a variety of neurological or metabolic abnormalities. Although frightening to the patient and family, most seizures are isolated and self-limited. The term *status epilepticus* is used only when a seizure lasts for more than thirty minutes or recurs at brief intervals during which the patient does not recover full consciousness. Parenteral benzodiazepines such as diazepam or lorazepam are effective in aborting active seizures. Antiepileptics such as phenytoin, phenobarbital, carbamazepine, valproic acid, and gabapentin can prevent future seizures. When the oral or intravenous route is not available, certain anticonvulsants can be given intramuscularly or rectally. Myoclonus, sometimes due to high doses of opioid analgesics, is often misinterpreted by patients and families as seizure activity.

Objectives

Attitudes/Behaviors

1. Defend supportive psychotherapy in the management of an adjustment disorder in the palliative care setting.

2. Describe possible family motivations for requesting assisted suicide for a terminally ill patient who lacks decision-making capacity.

3. Discuss the importance of using an interdisciplinary team approach when managing agitated terminal delirium in the home setting.

4. Compare the relative benefits and burdens of using physical restraints versus chemical restraints to manage agitation.

5. Defend a decision by a patient/family that may result in risk of injury for an agitated patient.

6. Discuss the meaning of a patient's non-disturbing visual hallucinations of deceased friends and relatives.

7. Explain the benefits and burdens of various approaches to diagnosing new-onset seizures in a terminally ill patient.

8. Understand the importance of recognizing and treating depression in terminally ill patients.

9. Defend the hospice and palliative medicine approach to caring for patients with advanced dementia.

10. Defend the process of evaluating a terminally ill patient with a diagnosis of delirium.

11. Describe the pertinence of a patient's psychosocial history to a differential diagnosis of depression.

Knowledge

1. Explain the differences between sadness, adjustment disorder, and depression.

2. List and define commonly encountered strategies for coping with advanced illness.

3. Summarize the psychological and physical symptoms of major depression.

4. Compare and contrast representative classes of antidepressant medications, including psychostimulants, selective serotonin-reuptake inhibitors (SSRIs), and tricyclic antidepressants.

5. Define delirium and contrast it with the definition of dementia.

6. List reversible causes of delirium which might be sought in patients with terminal illness.

7. Compare and contrast particular benzodiazepines with specific neuroleptic medications for control of delirium.

8. Summarize the benzodiazepines available for the management of anxiety and describe their advantages and disadvantages.

9. Describe indications for pharmacologic treatment of hallucinations.

10. Discuss specific alternative drugs and routes of drug delivery for benzodiazepines, neuroleptics, and antiepileptics.

11. Describe the management of extrapyramidal symptoms that may be encountered when using neuroleptic medications.

12. Describe the changes that occur in patients with end-stage dementia.

13. Describe a treatment plan that includes both pharmacologic and non-pharmocologic measures for a patient with dementia and reversed sleep-wake patterns.

Skills

1. Conduct a Folstein Mini-Mental Status Examination.

2. Explain a management plan for an acute change in mental status that includes a rationale for a change in the care setting.

3. Communicate effectively with a patient who is expressing suicidal ideation.

4. Describe alternatives for the medical management of the patient with recurrent seizures at home who is no longer able to take oral medications.

5. Treat the symptoms that occur with advanced dementia.

6. Differentiate among appropriate responses to advanced disease and depression.

7. Integrate at least three different approaches to the care of an anxious patient.

References

1. Bergevin P, Bergevin RM. Recognizing delirium in terminal patients. *Am J Hospice Palliat Care.* 196;13:28-9.
2. Breitbart W, Jacobsen PB. Psychiatric symptom management in terminal care. *Clin Geriatr Med.* 1996;12:329-47.
3. Cheng WC, Schuckers PL, Hauser G, et al. Psychosocial needs of family caregivers of terminally ill patients. *Psychol Rep.* 1994;75:1243-50.
4. deStoutz ND, Tapper M, Fainsinger RL. Reversible delirium in terminally ill patients. *J Pain Symptom Manage.* 1995;10:249-53.
5. Kurtz ME, Kurtz JC, Given CW, Given B. Predictors of postbereavement depressive symptomatology among family caregivers of cancer patients. *Support Care Cancer.* 1997;5:53-60.

6. Levy LJ, Derby JF, Martinkowski KS. Effects of membership in bereavement support groups on adaptation to conjugal bereavement. *Am J Community Psychol.* 1993;361-81.

7. Lipowski ZJ. Delirium in the elderly patient. *New Engl J Med.* 1989;320:578-581.

8. McGee EM. Can suicide intervention in hospice be ethical? *J Palliat Care.* 1997;13:27-33.

9. Doyle D, Hanks GWC, MacDonald N, eds. *Oxford Textbook of Palliative Medicine.* 2nd ed. New York: Oxford University Press; 1997.

10. Potter WZ, Rudorfer MV, Manji H. The pharmacologic treatment of depression. *New Engl J Med.* 1991;325:633-642.

11. Power D, Kelly S, Gilenan J, et al. Suitable screening tests for cognitive impairment and depression in the terminally ill—a prospective prevalence study. *Palliat Med.* 1993;7:213-18.

12. Roth AJ, Breitbart W. Psychiatric emergencies in terminally ill cancer patients. *Hematol Oncol Clin North Am.* 1996;10:235-59.

13. Rummans TA, Evans J, Krahn L and Flemin KC. Delirium in elderly patients: evaluation and management. *Mayo Clin Proc.* 1995;70:989-998.

14. Saunders C, Sykes N, eds. *The Management of Terminal Malignant Disease.* 3rd ed. Boston: Edward Arnold Publishers; 1993.

15. Truog RD, Berde CB, Mitchell C, Grier H. Barbiturates in the care of the terminally ill. *New Engl J Med.* 1992;327:1678-1682.

MODULE THIRTEEN

Hospice and Palliative Medicine for Pediatric Patients

Hospice and Palliative Care

Each year, over 85,000 children die in the United States. More than 50 percent of pediatric deaths occur in the neonatal period, due to prematurity or congenital anomalies. After one year of age, trauma is the leading cause of death, with a smaller number of children dying of chronic illnesses, including cancer and congenital, metabolic, or degenerative disorders.

The death of a child often is described as causing the deepest pain imaginable for loved ones. Frequently, the child's death results in significant feelings of guilt on the part of parents and siblings, and contributes to dysfunction in the entire family system. To ameliorate these adverse effects, a family-centered death should be encouraged whenever possible. Even when acute fatal conditions are managed in pediatric intensive and neonatal care units, palliative interventions and family involvement are important.

When a chronic illness is likely to result in childhood death, emotional support for the entire family should be provided throughout the child's life. Because the idea of a child dying is so aversive in our society, hospice and palliative care programs may need to serve as family advocates to ensure the child's physical and emotional suffering is acknowledged and carefully considered when making decisions about treatment. Such support can result in a healthier bereavement for the child's parents, grandparents, and siblings.

Often, hospice and palliative care programs can enrich the lives of all members of the family system.

The optimal time to begin comprehensive, family-oriented, child-centered care is at the time of diagnosis of a life-threatening condition. The following behaviors comprise the most effective approach to the care of dying children and their family members: acknowledging the seriousness of the illness, clarifying the child's and family's treatment goals, establishing a family care plan, providing continuity of care with the same team of caregivers, and recognizing the multidimensional nature of the child's and family's suffering. Families with terminally ill children often are young, with limited financial and emotional resources. Frequently, they feel abandoned by friends and family who, not knowing what to say or do, may avoid the family altogether.

Choice of words is particularly important when explaining palliative services to families. Families may reject the concept of hospice care because it connotes death and limited medical interventions. The terms "supportive care" or "palliative care" may be more acceptable because they suggest to families that they have done everything possible to save their child's life, while still ensuring the child's comfort.

Parents may need guidance to communicate effectively with their child about pain and suffering, and to recognize when the goal of cure is no longer reasonable. Hospice and palliative care staff can help attending physicians and the child's family clarify options, maximize the quality of the child's remaining time, support the child and family as the child's life draws to a close, improve symptom management, assist with grief work, and facilitate conflict resolution. With assistance from hospice and palliative care staff, families may decide to allow their child to die at home, which often diminishes the child's sense of isolation and allows siblings to participate in care. Participating in care is important for healthy bereavement, and often alleviates a sibling's sense of being alone, frightened, and uninformed.

Communication and Decision Making

Communication problems exacerbate the challenges associated with caring for a child with a life-limiting illness. Because children fear abandonment more than pain or death, they will endure significant suffering in silence to avoid alienating significant others. Play therapy and art therapy can be useful methods for facilitating communication with young children; however, specialized training may be needed to use them effectively.

Children's thought processes differ substantially from those of adults. Children think concretely; thus, euphemisms can be dangerous. Children are subject to finalism, that is, the belief that bad things happen to people when they are bad and being good protects people from bad things. Such beliefs distort a child's (and often an adult's) understanding of the causation of illness and may produce unacknowledged or unsuspected feelings of guilt. For children, admitting to having pain is the same as admitting they are bad. Thus, skilled communication is necessary when asking children about their thoughts and feelings. In addition, the egocentrism of children causes them to believe that everyone knows what they are thinking; thus, they may

not realize they have to communicate their thoughts verbally. Communication can be encouraged by soliciting children's opinions and clearly indicating to them that their ideas are important.

Practically and legally, some children have limited capacity to express their wishes regarding the goals of medical care. They must rely on parents, caregivers, or other responsible adults to interpret their needs and wishes. This responsibility can be overwhelming for parents. Futile medical interventions and unnecessary suffering may continue unabated because parents and other adults find it so difficult to discuss such issues with children and help them articulate their desires. Good communication and realistic, factual information are the keys to appropriate care.

The inherently difficult process of making treatment decisions for children with poor prognoses is further hampered by the Baby Doe regulations, which are widely misunderstood by medical personnel. The Baby Doe regulations, which impact the federal supplementation of state Child Protective Services funds only, require the continuation of life-sustaining treatment for all infants under the age of one year, regardless of projected quality of life, unless the infant is imminently dying or permanently comatose. In addition, when a life-threatening condition is irreversible, treatment is *not* required—an exception that many healthcare professionals fail to understand. Hospice and palliative care could serve as appropriate alternatives.

No legal mechanism exists for honoring the autonomy of children under the age of 15. Often, the wishes of more mature children are unsolicited or ignored, despite the fact that many chronically ill children have remarkably mature views of illness and death.

The availability of new technologies, transplants, ECMO, protease inhibitors, and liquid ventilation further confuse the decision-making process. Lacking experience with such interventions, parents and children cannot assess the relative benefits and burdens of treatments. Physicians commonly present only the positive side of technical interventions, making it even more difficult for parents and children to make informed decisions. Thus, it is imperative for physicans to present both the benefits and burdens of treatment options, to offer palliative care as a treatment option, and to encourage parents and children to partici-pate in the decision-making process, to the extent they desire and are able to do so. When patients and families are struggling with the decision-making process, physicians should provide guidance by recommending a course of action and explaining why it is likely to be the best option for a particular situation.

Hospice and palliative care personnel should ensure the child's wishes are consid-ered when making important decisions about medical care. Regardless of age, children should be allowed discretion and autonomy consistent with their maturity and degree of understanding. Even toddlers can exert control over which hand will have the IV or which loved one will remain in the room during procedures. Older children can deter-mine the timing of and need for conscious sedation and make other procedure-related decisions.

Appropriate planning requires encouraging children to discuss their feelings and concep-tions of suffering, which are rarely volun-teered. Children should also be encouraged to participate in family meetings when treat-ments and prognosis are summarized. No other person can adequately represent the child's point of view.

The Child's Perspective

Children's wishes regarding care are shaped by their stage of development. Infants and pre-schoolers want love and affection from their families, who must always be near. School-age children often want anything that will allow them to return to school, to be with friends, and to learn. Because older teenagers realize their opportunities to experience the benefits and responsibilities of adulthood are

slipping away, they may wish to get married, graduate early from high school, try new activities, stay with friends, or live alone. By providing excellent symptom management and facilitating communication, hospice and palliative care programs can help ensure important goals are attained.

Without ever being told, even very young children (as young as three years old) know when they are seriously and/or terminally ill. Denial and pretense only cause children to lose trust in adults and feel more frightened. Children are not born with concepts or fears about death. Their conceptions of death begin with early infantile fears of separation from the warmth and smell of familiar caretakers, and gradually evolve to more existential constructs. When communicating with seri-ously ill or bereaved children about death and dying, the developmental stages described below should be considered. However, age ranges should be used only as guidelines—a child's illness experiences and intelligence can considerably alter the developmental under-standing of death. Faulkner describes four major developmental phases:

- **Separation** (age 0-3, Sensorimotor - Piaget). Children do not distinguish death from abandonment; they need close physical contact to allay anxiety.
- **Structural** (age 3-6, Preoperational). Death is reversible. Magical thinking and egocentrism lead children to believe they may have caused their own illness or that of a loved one. Children in this phase believe that only old people die; they cannot conceive of their own deaths. The most effective methods for allaying anxiety and fear are to communicate directly with children about their views of the problem, provide as much physical contact as the child desires, and offer age-appropriate factual explanations and reassurance.
- **Functional** (age 6-12, Concrete operations). In this phase, a child's logical thought processes are more developed. As abstract thinking develops, children who are seven

and older can usually comprehend the four components of death: irreversibility (dead organisms cannot reanimate); universality (all living things die); nonfunctionality (dead organisms do not eat or move); and causality (death is caused by illness or trauma, not by bad thoughts). In this phase, children benefit from factual information, from retaining as much control as possible, and from access to nonverbal means of communication, for example, drawing, dance, and play therapy.

- **Abstract** (over 12, Formal operations). Older children can appreciate the broader ramifications of death and dying on society at large. Body image and peer support are of paramount importance. Grief may be manifested by acting out behavior. A heightened sense of tragedy and emotional sensitivity are common and can be usefully channeled into making tapes and mementos for soon-to-be bereaved family and friends. Providing firm love, support, and as much independence as possible usually benefits adolescent children.

The Family's Perspective

Families often resist hospice or palliative care for their children. Because it is difficult both for family members and physicians to acknowledge a child's life-threatening condition, families may reject the standard hospice philosophy, in particular the phrase, *terminally ill*. They may also refuse to sign orders not to resuscitate or to forgo therapies that might become available in the future. Medical uncertainty regarding prognostication can disqualify children from receiving hospice services. Acknowledging the need for a flexible approach to care may be the only way to gain a family's trust and an opportunity to provide much-needed palliative care for children with life-threatening conditions.

Families with profoundly ill children need education, emotional support, and practical assistance. Parents usually want to perform as

much of the caregiving as possible. They need to feel confident about managing symptoms at home and allowing their child to die peacefully in familiar surroundings instead of in a hospital. Respite from the responsibilities of caregiving, whether for a few hours or a few days, may be greatly needed. Help from hospice volunteers with mundane chores and with the care and amusement of siblings is often appreciated.

Support groups can benefit some families by decreasing their sense of isolation and helping dispel misconceptions about certain topics, such as communicating with children. Social workers can assist not only with counseling, but also with issues such as loss of income due to one parent remaining home, funeral arrangements, talking with siblings about death, and informing the school and community about the child's condition and ultimate demise. Siblings often suffer from lack of parental attention and may exhibit anger, jealousy, guilt, and doubts about self-worth. Hospice and palliative care staff can talk with siblings about such issues and help parents understand the sibling's responses, averting unnecessary conflicts.

The Caregivers' and Institutions' Perspective

Many hospice and palliative care workers are reluctant to care for children with life-limiting illnesses because they fear over-identification and potential emotional distress when the child dies. However, after caring for a terminally ill child, the majority of staff report a deep sense of satisfaction. Due to the likelihood of close identification with an ill child, caregivers must set appropriate limits on their involvement to ensure the family retains control over the child's care, with help as needed from team members.

In most cases, parents rely on the knowledge and competence of their physicians. However, few physicians and other healthcare professionals receive adequate training in pediatric pain and symptom management. Special training should be provided to physicians and other caregivers to ensure they understand the special needs of pediatric patients. Parents with long-term experience dealing with a chronically ill child may have become experts themselves, in which case they often need little more than validation of their skills.

Due to limitations in reimbursement mechanisms, most hospice care for children is provided without compensation. When children are admitted to hospice programs without a certification of terminal illness (a prognosis of six months or less, if the disease runs it normal course), the services rendered are not reimbursable under most states' Medicaid Hospice Benefits. Non-governmental insurers may not offer a hospice benefit for children; if one exists, it frequently mimics the Medicare/Medicaid requirements.

Hospice programs with home health agency licenses may receive reimbursement for medical services for terminally ill children, but pastoral care, social services, and art or music therapy are rarely covered. Smaller hospice programs may be reluctant to care for pediatric patients due to lack of reimbursement for the resource-intensive services required by dying children and their families. Larger hospice programs can sometimes provide services by sponsoring fund-raising campaigns to support hospice care for pediatric patients.

In England, the provision of long-term hospice and pediatric palliative care is common. Free-standing children's hospices offering respite care are increasingly available. In England, the majority of pediatric hospice patients suffer from progressive neurodegenerative or neuromuscular disorders. In the United States, most hospices adhere to Medicaid criteria; thus, they are more likely to receive reimbursement for the care of children with end-stage leukemia, other advanced cancers, or AIDS. In many cases, children are admitted for hospice care only during the last days of life.

Common Life-Limiting Conditions in Children

Acquired immunodeficiency syndrome (AIDS): The incidence of acquired immunodeficiency syndrome is increasing among the heterosexual population, leading to increases in infant AIDS. AIDS is the sixth leading cause of death in the 0-4 year-old age group, and the seventh leading cause in the 5-14 year-old age group. In the United States, approximately 6,000 children are born annually to women infected with HIV. Among HIV-infected women who were not treated with zidovudine (Retrovir) during pregnancy, transmission of HIV occurs in 25 percent of births. Transmission of HIV decreases dramatically when women are treated with zidovudine (Retrovir) during pregnancy.

Most studies describe two distinct courses of illness in HIV-infected children. Approximately 16 percent to 33 percent of children experience unremitting illness, often with a component of neurodegeneration. They develop AIDS at a median age of four months, with death occurring at four years of age, on average. However, most perinatally infected children exhibit no or minor manifestations until they are older (median time to AIDS is 6.1 years), with death occurring approximately three years after an AIDS diagnosis. The future impact of protease inhibitors and other antiretroviral medications on childhood AIDS is unknown.

Caring for children with AIDS is very challenging, due in part to the high incidence of associated pain syndromes. In addition, the mother is virtually always infected and the father, when present, may also be infected, as may some of the siblings. Families may be financially unstable, with little or no extended family support, and parents may be unreliable caregivers.

Hereditary disorders and congenital anomalies: Hereditary disorders and congenital developmental anomalies, including diseases with metabolic defects (e.g., Tay

Sachs) can cause significant emotional pain, anger, and guilt among parents and grandparents. Because hereditary diseases may not be obvious until after several children are born, some families have several affected children and experience multiple childhood deaths. Although developmental anomalies are unlikely to recur within a family, the mother is sometimes blamed (silently or out loud, by self or others) for causing the problem due to real or imagined prenatal indiscretions. This issue must be explored and defused.

Persistent vegetative state (PVS): Patients with PVS should be considered for palliative care because it is a life-threatening condition even when all available medical treatments are provided. In adults and older teens, the average life expectancy from time of onset of PVS is nine years. Life expectancy is shorter when onset occurs at a younger age. Infantile onset of PVS is associated with an average life expectancy of 2.6 years.

Pediatric malignancies: The overall cure rate of pediatric malignancies is 66.2 percent. The most common pediatric malignancy, acute lymphocytic leukemia (ALL), comprises approximately one third of pediatric cancer diagnoses and has a cure rate >80 percent. Thus, when a child dies of this form of cancer, the family's sense of failure may be magnified. Brain tumors are the next most frequently diagnosed cancer among children; these have a more dismal prognosis. Lymphoma occurs in approximately 10 percent of cases and is curable 60 percent to 90 percent of the time.

Pediatric Pain Management

Pain and symptom assessment and management in pediatric populations can be quite difficult. As recently as the 1980s, widespread misconceptions existed concerning children's ability to perceive pain. It is now clear that children perceive pain, even in utero. In fact, studies have shown that pain inhibition pathways are less developed in infants and young children, resulting in increased transmission of pain stimuli to the brain when compared with older children.

The principles of pain management in children are similar to those in adults, though dosages are different. Assessment techniques should be tailored to the child's developmental stage. Opioids are safe and effective for the treatment of pediatric pain. Respiratory depression is rare, and opioid clearance differs only in the very young (< 3 months) or premature. Titration, treatment of breakthrough pain, and the weaning of children from opioids are accomplished in the same manner as with adults.

Medical professionals caring for pediatric patients who undergo acute care interventions must serve as advocates for aggressive prevention and treatment of pain. As with adult patients, some physicians inappropriately withhold analgesics due to ignorance of the adverse effects of uncontrolled pain, lack of knowledge about appropriate and effective use of opioids, misconceptions about a child's appreciation of pain, and other pain-related matters.

Infants react to pain with prolonged, loud crying, diffuse motor activity, and characteristic facial grimaces, for example, furrowed brows, increased nasolabial folds, and a taut, cupped tongue. A smaller percentage of infants (20%) respond to pain with decreased movement. Toddlers exhibit anticipatory distress, verbal protestations, and attempts at protective withdrawal. As children understand the need for invasive procedures, their behavioral manifestations of distress decrease markedly, indicating either an acculturation to expected responses or decreased appreciation of pain due to cognitive amelioration of the sensation.

Children define pain according to their developmental levels. Young children are perceptually dominated and describe what they can see as being the most painful, which explains why preschool children become so anxious when a small scratch produces bleeding. Early school-age children describe pain in context and understand its impact on mood. Older children understand pain in more universal and existential terms, as do adults.

Correcting a child's misconceptions about pain is very important. Because young children perceive pain as punishment, they must be reassured that they are good people and have done nothing to deserve pain.

Because children often have fertile imaginations, complementary therapies such as distraction, music, relaxation, or hypnosis are useful adjuncts to local anesthetics during procedures. However, such therapies usually should not be used as substitutes for scrupulous pharmacologic pain control.

Children react to pain in many of the same ways as adults. Children with chronic pain tend to protect painful areas and move very little. They may seem apathetic or whiny. Such behaviors change dramatically when their pain is relieved.

Hospice and palliative care staff frequently ask children to rate their pain. Very young children have limited quantification skills but do understand the concept of little, medium and big. As children mature, more refined methods for measuring pain can be used, including the Hester poker chips tool, the Eland color tool, the faces pain scale, and numeric pain scales. Children also communicate about pain through drawings and behavior.

In children, pain is most often treatment related, that is, caused by invasive procedures or the side effects of medications. Treatment-related pain includes mucositis pain (often severe enough to require opioid analgesics), neuropathic pain related to chemotherapeutic agents, and pain related to surgery or bone marrow biopsies.

Because pain is so often treatment-related, much of the pain children experience is preventable. Local anesthetics such as EMLA combined with conscious sedation or brief opioid analgesia (such as with transmucosal fentanyl citrate) should be used liberally. It is crucial to prevent pain with the use of cutaneous application local anesthetics for IV insertions, portacath entries, lumbar punctures, and other invasive procedures. Before anxiety-provoking procedures are attempted, children should receive instruction in distraction techniques and, when needed, conscious sedation should be used.

The prolonged, progressive, localized pain so common in adults with cancer is rare in children, due in part to the types of malignancies they experience. Children experience a higher proportion of hematologic malignancies, and progress rapidly to death when the disease cannot be controlled. Disease-related pain most often occurs in the bones and bone marrow and is diffuse; therefore, radiation therapy and nerve blocks are less helpful than for adults. Pain may be localized within the central nervous system, related to primary brain tumors, carcinomatous meningitis, and spinal cord compression.

AIDS-associated pain is very common and poorly understood. It may be related to skin and esophageal lesions, other infections, or organomegaly, or it may be neuropathic in origin. Headaches are common. Pediatric AIDS specialists may neglect the treatment of pain while they are addressing numerous other issues associated with childhood AIDS. However, children should not be expected to live with pain. Medical professionals must emphasize pain control as a significant quality-of-life issue.

Children under five years old generally cannot swallow pills. Many medications either do not come in liquid form or the liquid formulation tastes awful. Oncologists and AIDS specialists prefer that medications not be administered per rectum; in any case, most children do not like suppositories. Because many chronically ill children already have either a central venous line or a gastrostomy tube, medications often can be administered using these routes. Patient-controlled analgesia pumps have been successfully used with children as young as four years old.

Non-Pain Symptoms

Very few studies have investigated non-pain symptoms in children. The same types of symptoms are reported as those experienced by adults, but they may occur at different rates. Suggested therapies are similar to those for adults, with doses modified appropriately.

Summary

Hospice and palliative care for children living with life-limiting conditions is appropriate and effective. In its absence, symptom management may receive inadequate attention and potentially harmful therapy may be continued. When helping children with life-limiting conditions, the role of hospice and palliative programs differs from that with adults. Caregivers must engage in active, facilitative, and dynamic interactions with physicians and families. Hospice and palliative care programs cannot wait for the families of terminally ill children to approach them; the few children who are referred for hospice and palliative care are likely to arrive so late in the illness trajectory that the benefits of such care will be unrealized.

Hospice and palliative care programs must establish partnerships with other components of the healthcare system, thus allowing children with life-limiting conditions and their families access to much-needed symptom control and emotional and spiritual support. Only then can hospice and palliative programs enrich the lives of terminally ill children and their families.

Objectives

Attitudes/Behaviors

1. Describe treatment goals for children with life-limiting conditions and the differences between curative and palliative treatments.

2. Defend the importance of providing hospice and palliative care for dying children as an active, desirable, and valuable service to dying children, their families, caregivers, and society.

3. Discuss the reality of pediatric death as part of the natural life cycle, though such deaths seem premature.

4. Describe the need for skilled communication when discussing death and dying with children, their families, and caregivers.

5. Describe common contributors to suffering experienced by children with life-limiting conditions.

6. Identify personal and societal conflicts and anxieties about childhood death which may interfere with the provision of pediatric palliative care.

7. Discuss the impact of cultural and religious practices and beliefs on the care of dying children.

8. Recognize the importance of providing emotional and spiritual support for everyone involved in the direct care of the terminally ill child, especially siblings, grandparents, extended relatives, and friends.

9. Discuss the need for education of pediatric medical caregivers regarding pediatric palliative and hospice services.

10. Describe the importance of developing relationships among hospice and palliative care programs and the tertiary care centers that serve their catchment area.

11. Outline why hospice and palliative care must be offered to children in the intensive care setting.

12. Defend the practice of allowing children to participate in decision making during the course of their illness.

13. Defend the aggressive treatment of pain in children with life-limiting conditions.

14. Describe the need for pediatric palliative and hospice care.

Knowledge

1. Describe differences in hospice care for children (infants, children and adolescents) and adults, in terms of admission requirements and family and physician dynamics.

2. Describe the Baby Doe regulations and their influence on medical decision making.

3. Discuss developmental influences on the average child's understanding of death.

4. Discuss the determinants of a child's capacity to make health care decisions.

5. List diagnoses that should lead to consideration of hospice or palliative care for children.

6. Outline the role of palliative care for a child with a potentially life-limiting condition.

7. Discuss emotional, legal, and ethical factors influencing the decision-making process for children with potentially life-threatening conditions.

8. Describe effective methods for communicating about death and dying with children at various developmental stages.

9. Describe differences in pain perception between young children and adults.

10. Explain techniques for assessing pain in children of varying ages.

11. Describe common life-limiting illnesses in the pediatric population, and their usual disease course.

Skills

1. Assess, treat, and manage all types of pain in infants, children, and adolescents.

2. Communicate effectively with dying children and their families to ensure informed decisions are made when planning end-of-life care.

3. Manage physical and emotional contributors to suffering effectively.

4. Communicate effectively with other healthcare professionals to ensure a dying child is carefully attended and optimal comfort measures are provided.

5. Assure a dying child, family, and caregivers that they will not be abandoned and exhibit behavior that supports the assurance.

6. Encourage as much patient control as possible during all phases of a terminal pediatric illness.

7. Educate other healthcare professionals about the opportunities for interpersonal growth that occur when caring for children with life-limiting conditions.

8. Assess, treat, and manage all types of non-pain symptoms experienced by infants, children, and adolescents.

References

1. Anand KJS, Hickey PR. Pain and its effects on the human neonate and fetus. *N Engl J Med.* 1987;317:1321-9.
2. Ashwal S, Perkin RW, Orr R. When too much is not enough. *Pediatr Ann.* 1992;21(5):311-14, 316-7.
3. Barnhart HX, et al. Natural history of human immunodeficiency virus disease in perinatally infected children: an analysis from the Pediatric Spectrum of Disease Project. *Pediatrics.* 1996; 97(5):710-716.
4. Bartholome WG. A new understanding of consent in pediatric practice: consent, parental permission and child assent. *Pediatr Ann.* 1989;18(4):262-5.
5. Black D. Bereavement. In: Goldman A, ed. *Care of the Dying Child.* Oxford: Oxford University Press; 1994.
6. Bluebond-Langner M. *The Private Worlds of Dying Children.* Princeton, NJ: Princeton University Press; 1978.
7. Boyd-Franklin N, Steiner GL, Boland MG. *Children, Families and HIV/AIDS; Psychosocial and Therapeutic Issues.* New York: The Guilford Press; 1995: 20.
8. Brown JM, O'Keefe J, Sanders SH, Baker B. Developmental changes in children's cognition to stressful and painful situations. *J Pediatr Psychol.* 1986;11:343-57.
9. Collins JJ, Greake J, Grier HE, et al. Patient-controlled analgesia for mucositis pain in children: a three-period crossover study comparing morphine and hydromorphone. *J Pediatrics.* 1996; 129:722-728.
10. Committee on Bioethics, American Academy of Pediatrics. Informed consent, parental permission and assent in pediatric practice. *Pediatrics.* 1995;95(2):314-976.
11. Committee on Bioethics, American Academy of Pediatrics. Guidelines on forgoing life-sustaining medical treatment. *Pediatrics.* 1994;93(3):532-6.
12. Devereux JA, Jones DPH, Dickenson DL. Can children withhold consent to treatment? *BMJ.* 1993;306:1459-61.
13. Doyal L, Henning P. Stopping treatment for end-stage renal failure: the rights of children and adolescents. *J Pediatr Nephrol.* 1994;8:768-91.
14. Faulkner KW. Children's understanding of death. In: Dailey AA, Goltzer SG. *Hospice Care for Children.* New York: Oxford University Press; 1993.
15. Fitzgerald M, Koltzenburg M. The functional development of descending inhibitory pathways in the dorsolateral funiculus of the newborn rat spinal cord. *Dev Brain Research.* 1983;265:1-9.
16. Foot ABM. The changing face of paediatric oncology. *Palliat Med.* 1995;9:193-9.
17. Freyer DR. Children with cancer: special considerations in the discontinuation of life sustaining treatment. *J Med Pediatr Oncol.* 1992;20:136-42.
18. Gardner P, Hudson BL. Advance report of final mortality statistics. 1993 *Mon Vital Stat Rep.* 1996:44(Suppl), No. 7.
19. King NMP, Cross AW. Children as decision-makers: guidelines for pediatricians. *J Pediatrics.* 1989;115(1):10-16.
20. Koren G. Informed consent in pediatric research. In: *Textbook of Ethics in Pediatric Research.* Malabar, Fla: Krieger Publishing Co; 1993.

21. Kriel RL, Krach LE, Jones-Saete C, et al. Outcome of children with prolonged unconsciousness and vegetative state. *Pediatr Neurol.* 1993:9(5):362-8.
22. Kubler-Ross E. *On Children and Death.* New York: Macmillan Publishing Co; 1983.
23. Lansdown R. Communicating with children. In: Goldman A. *Caring for the Dying Child.* New York: Oxford University Press; 1994:102.
24. Lauer ME, Mulhern RK, Schell MJ, Camitta BM. Long-term follow-up of parental adjustment following a child's death at home or in the hospital. *Cancer.* 1989;63:988-994.
25. Lantos JD, Tyson JE, Allen A, et al. Withholding and withdrawing life sustaining medical treatment in neonatal intensive care: issues for the 1990's. *Arch Dis Child.* 1994:71:F218-23.
26. Leikin S. The role of adolescents in decisions concerning their cancer therapy. *Cancer.* 1993; 71 suppl:3342-6.
27. Martinson IM. Improving care of dying children. *West J Med.* 1995:163:258-62.
28. Miser JS, Miser AW. Pain and symptom control. In: Dailey AA. *Hospice Care for Children.* New York: Oxford University Press; 1993.
29. *Monthly Vital Statistics Report.* US Dept. of Health and Human Services, CDC and Prevention, National Center for Health Statistics. 1996;45 (suppl 2):15. Table 9.
30. Nelson LJ. Forgoing treatment of critically ill newborns and the legal legacy of Baby Doe. *Clin Ethics Report.* 1992;6(2):1-6.
31. Novelli VM. Assessing prognosis in infant infected with human immunodeficiency virus. *Pediatrics.* 1996;129(5):623-5.
32. President's Commission for the Study of Ethical Problems in Medicine and Biomedical and Behavioral Research. *Deciding to Forgo Life-Sustaining Treatment: A Report on the Ethical, Medical and Legal Issues in Treatment Decisions.* Washington, DC: Government Printing Office; 1987.
33. Rothenberg KH, et al., eds. *Biolaw: A Legal & Ethical Report on Medical, Health Care and Bioengineering.* Vol. 1. Frederick, Md: University Publications of America; 1986.
34. Sanchez E, Paya J. Estimating HIV vertical transmission: a meta-analytic approach. Presented at the VIII International Congress on AIDS/III STD World Congress. Amsterdam, July, 1992.
35. Schechter NL, Allen DA, Hanson K. Status of pediatric pain control: a comparison of hospital analgesic usage in children and adults. *Pediatrics.* 1986;77:11-15.
36. Silverman WA. A hospice setting for humane neonatal death. *Pediatrics.* 1982;69(2):239-40.
37. Susman EJ, Hersh SP, Nannis ED, et al. Conceptions of cancer: the perspectives of child and adolescent patients and their families. *J Pediatr Psychiat.* 1982;7(3):253-61.
38. Stahlman M. Presidential address, American Pediatric Society: medical ethics and the law. *Pediatr Res.* 1986;20(9): 913-4.
39. Tyson J. Evidence-based ethics and the care of premature infants. *Future Child.* 1995;5(1):197-213.

Hospice and Palliative Medicine for Patients with HIV Disease

Challenges Associated with Palliation of HIV Disease

Patients with human immunodeficiency virus (HIV) disease present multiple challenges for hospice and palliative medicine physicians and other healthcare providers. Such challenges include providing effective treatments for opportunistic infections, dispelling misconceptions about the goals of prophylaxis and treatment, and ensuring continuity of care despite the typically episodic nature of managing patients with HIV disease.

Although patients with HIV disease experience acute, chronic, and terminal phases of illness, palliation is necessary throughout the entire illness continuum. Many of the manifestations of HIV disease, such as neuropathy, are best treated symptomatically from their inception. The benefits of palliative care should not be reserved just for the last few weeks or days of a patient's life.

As with most chronic illnesses, appropriate therapy focuses on disease-specific treatments. When the illness progresses, disease-specific palliative interventions are directed at opportunistic illnesses, such as mycobacterium tuberculosis, Kaposi's sarcoma, or cytomegalovirus retinitis.

Misconceptions about the goals of standard, disease-specific therapies for palliating certain opportunistic illness associated with HIV have caused confusion among some hospice providers and insurers. Hospice programs may deny admission to patients receiving prophylaxis and treatment to prevent or lessen symptoms of opportunistic infections. Such *a priori* limits on care are based on misunderstandings about the nature of palliative treatments and the goals of care for patients with HIV disease, and should be carefully reviewed.

To palliate the multiple sources of suffering associated with HIV disease, for example, physical, psychosocial, emotional, and spiritual distress, physicians should apply the principles of palliative medicine throughout the entire continuum of the patient's illness. Patients with HIV disease may also experience additional suffering caused by treatments themselves, for example, the initiation of antiretroviral therapy. Some therapies for opportunistic infections are associated with anorexia, nausea, vomiting, diarrhea, headache, fatigue, and neuropathy. Physicians should anticipate adverse effects and initiate appropriate palliative therapies as needed.

Ideally, a palliative regimen is consistent with the patient's goals of therapy, treats discomfort and distressing symptoms effectively, is easy to administer, and is associated with a minimum of adverse effects. The efficacy of palliative therapies should be continually reassessed, especially during the final days of a patient's life, when intense focus is placed on maintaining comfort and controlling symptoms.

Management of Opportunistic Infections

Opportunistic infections (OIs) respond variably to treatment and prophylaxis. At one end of the spectrum are infections such as pneumocystis carinii pneumonia (PCP), which generally respond well to treatment with simple, efficacious, prophylactic regimens. At the other end of the spectrum are infections such as mycobacterium avium complex (MAC), which are difficult to treat because they require simultaneous administration of multiple antibiotics. Until recently, MAC prophylaxis also was associated with numerous adverse effects. Instead of discussing the many therapeutic options for each OI (see reference # 2: CDC guidelines for treatment and prophylaxis of OIs), this section discusses four opportunistic infections and presents palliative regimens for their management that illustrate the principles of disease-specific palliation.

Pneumocystis Carinii Pneumonia

Due to the widespread use of prophylaxis, pneumocystis carinii pneumonia (PCP) is causing fewer deaths among patients with HIV disease. Acute PCP usually responds to trimethoprim-sulfamethoxazole (TMP-SMZ), or pentamidine in sulfa allergic patients. Primary or secondary prophylaxis of PCP is generally achieved with one double strength TMP-SMZ tablet daily. This regimen also offers protection against toxoplasmic encephalitis. For sulfa-allergic patients, dapsone is a reasonable alternative.

These prophylactic treatment regimens are effective, well tolerated, and easily administered, and provide excellent symptom control for patients with moderately advanced and end-stage HIV disease. When patients object to the therapies or are unable to tolerate them, PCP-associated dyspnea, fever, and generalized discomfort can be treated with morphine, oxygen, acetaminophen, nonsteroidal anti-inflammatory drugs (NSAIDs) or prednisone. However, no traditional palliative regimens are as effective as TMP-SMZ or dapsone-pyrimethamine for treating symptoms associated with PCP.

Cryptococcal Meningitis

The hallmarks of cryptococcal meningitis are severe headache and fever. Though impossible to eradicate, acute cryptococcosis responds best to amphotericin and flucytosine, followed by lifelong suppressive therapy with an azole antifungal medication.

Although primary prophylaxis of cryptococcosis is not widely recommended, secondary prophylaxis with oral fluconazole or itraconazole is approximately 97 percent effective in preventing recurrence of acute meningitis or systemic cryptococcosis. Weekly doses of intravenous amphotericin effectively suppress recurrent cryptococcal infections in patients with azole-resistant infection. Amphotericin requires intravenous access but it is generally well tolerated and also provides prophylaxis against oral and esophageal candidiasis.

The effectiveness and ease of administration of these cryptococcal-suppressing interventions make them excellent palliative regimens for most patients. By contrast, when cryptococcus is left untreated, strong analgesics are necessary to treat the persistent headache of cryptococcal meningitis, and may produce unwanted side effects. Many of the adverse side effects can be ameliorated with other medications, but suppressive treatment is more easily administered, and provides better symptom relief with fewer untoward effects.

Cytomegalovirus Retinitis

In patients with < 50 CD4 cells/ul, cytomegalovirus (CMV) causes esophageal ulcers, enteritis, and systemic symptoms. However, the most disabling and disturbing manifestation of CMV is retinitis, which causes progressive blindness. Understandably, prevention of blindness is a high priority for HIV patients with CMV.

Generally, CMV retinitis is treated acutely with intravenous ganciclovir, foscarnet, or cidofovir. After acute therapy, options for suppression include continued, less-intensive intravenous therapy, oral ganciclovir, intravitreal ganciclovir, foscarnet or cidofovir, or intraocular sustained-release ganciclovir implants. The oral and intravenous secondary regimens are reasonably effective in preventing systemic manifestations of CMV, as well as the development of CMV retinitis in the contralateral eye.

Although none of these regimens is 100 percent effective, they represent the best opportunity for preserving sight. Various studies report progression of retinitis in approximately 15 days without treatment, versus approximately 60 days with intravenous treatment and 226 days with ganciclovir implants. However, the intravenous and intraocular regimens are invasive and expensive, and the oral regimen entails taking many pills daily. The applicability of these regimens may be limited by cost and by the patient's physical and psychological acceptance of treatment.

For people dying of HIV disease, the prospect of going blind in the final days, weeks, or months of life is very disturbing. Although not totally effective, the incomplete benefits provided by the above regimens seem justified because they offer patients the best chance of preserving sight. Prevention is the best available palliation of blindness.

Mycobacterium Avium Complex

In patients with < 100 CD4 cells/ul, disseminated mycobacterium avium complex (MAC) infection tends to cause fevers, weight loss, diarrhea, anemia, and other cytopenias. The standard treatment for MAC disease is associated with a number of problems, making it a poor choice for palliative therapy. In non-palliative care settings, MAC is usually

treated with three or four antibiotics, often requiring four to six administrations of medication daily. The medications cause several adverse side effects, most notably cytopenias, abnormalities of liver function, nausea, abdominal pain, and anorexia. More importantly, the standard treatment with multiple medications incompletely relieves the systemic symptoms of MAC. The burdens imposed by suboptimal efficacy, poor tolerability, and difficult administration are likely to outweigh the benefits of standard MAC therapy for patients with end-stage HIV disease.

For patients with end-stage HIV disease, palliation of MAC disease usually is best achieved with a combination of antidiarrheals, acetaminophen, and NSAIDS. Cholestyramine powder can be effective for diarrhea refractory to diphenoxylate-atropine and loperamide. Recent data show that primary prophylaxis with azithromycin, 1200 mg weekly, is effective in preventing systemic MAC disease. Often, this simple treatment is well tolerated, making it a reasonable palliative therapy in end-stage HIV disease, when symptom prevention is the primary goal.

HIV-Associated Cancers

With the notable exception of Kaposi's sarcoma, palliation of many HIV-associated cancers follows the traditional model for treating other cancers. Assessments of the efficacy of palliative interventions for HIV-associated cancer should be based on the treatment's acceptability to the patient, side effects, ease of administration, and effectiveness of symptom relief.

Kaposi's Sarcoma

In patients with HIV disease, Kaposi's sarcoma (KS) manifests as mucocutaneous and visceral lesions. KS can appear relatively early in the course of HIV disease, before patients exhibit other signs of immunocompromise. KS responds to several chemotherapeutic regimens, including adriamycin, vincristine, vinblastine, bleomycin, or liposomal doxorubicin/daunorubicin. Radiation therapy is effective for treating localized KS lesions. New treatments for KS are in continual development and testing. The distribution of KS lesions and the patient's acceptance and tolerance of therapy are important factors when choosing the best method of palliation.

Many of the manifestations of mucocutaneous KS (e.g., bulky oral and facial lesions, rectal lesions and ulcers, and lesions on the trunk, extremities, and genitals that cause edema and pain) are best palliated using the above standard therapies. These chemotherapeutic regimens can be administered every two weeks and tend to be well tolerated. Hematologic toxicities should be anticipated and, if indicated, treated with dose reductions or hematologic growth factors. Visceral KS also responds to systemic therapy.

Focal cutaneous KS lesions and pulmonary KS respond to radiation therapy; however, treating oral KS with radiation causes relatively severe mucosal reactions, even at low doses. Some radiation therapists caution against radiation of KS-involved lymph nodes because of the risk of decreased lymphatic drainage secondary to radiation-induced scarring and obstruction.

Primary Central Nervous System Lymphoma

Primary central nervous system lymphoma (PCNSL) occurs more frequently in patients with HIV disease than in the general population. Unfortunately, PCNSL is very aggressive and responds poorly to disease-specific therapy. Although approximately 75 percent of patients initially respond to radiation therapy, most experience early recurrence of the cancer. Average survival is two to three months post diagnosis.

Palliation of PCNSL usually follows the model employed with other cancers. Aggressive radiation therapy is directed at tumor

shrinkage. When irreversible recurrence or metastasis occurs, traditional palliative methods are appropriate, for example, glucocorticoids, anti-seizure medications, and analgesics. Recurrences are much less responsive to radiation.

Systemic Manifestations of HIV Disease

The systemic manifestations of HIV disease include pain, gastrointestinal distress, weight loss, depression, and fatigue. While some of these symptoms are managed as they would be in any other illness, some require more selective therapy.

Neuropathic Pain

Neuropathic pain commonly occurs in patients with HIV disease. Typical causes of neuropathy in patients with HIV disease include HIV-associated sensory polyneuropathy, acute and post-herpetic neuralgia, CMV neuropathy, and nucleoside toxicity (ddI, ddC, d4T). Neuropathic pain is distinguished from visceral and somatic pain by its characteristic burning, tingling, and electrical sensations; it usually responds to treatment with tricyclic antidepressants (TCAs), anticonvulsants, or steroids. Once a maximally tolerated dose of a TCA is achieved, anticonvulsants may be added for increased efficacy. Generally, these agents are started at the same doses as for seizure control. The principles of selection and titration parallel those for TCAs.

Depression

Depression is common among people with HIV disease, affecting as many as 30 percent of patients during the course of their illness. Selective serotonin reuptake inhibitors (SSRIs) are effective for treating depression; generally, they are well tolerated and can be dosed once a day. TCAs remain viable choices for the treatment of depression, especially if they are already being used to treat neuropathy. Combining an SSRI and a TCA may precipitate serotonin syndrome, characterized by tachycardia, flushing, hypertension, and diarrhea due to decreased metabolism of the TCA. However, in resistant cases, the patient's clinical condition may warrant an appropriate combination trial.

Diarrhea

Diarrhea is usually palliated effectively in patients with end-stage HIV disease without undertaking a diagnostic evaluation. Over-the-counter agents such as loperamide and diphenoxylate-atropine are useful when titrated to effect. These agents contain weak opioid derivatives that slow gastrointestinal motility and affect water and electrolyte movement throughout the bowel. For patients with intractable diarrhea, deodorized tincture of opium and other opiate agents can be titrated with excellent results. Bulk-forming and resin-binding agents can be very effective treatments for diarrhea, but they should be used with caution because of the risk of fecal impaction from inadequate fluid intake. Octreotide, a synthetic somatostatin analogue with a variety of gastrointestinal effects, has been effective in treating diarrhea approximately 50 to 60 percent of the time. The major disadvantages of octreotide are its high cost and the need for subcutaneous administration on a regular basis.

Antiretroviral Therapy in End-Stage HIV

Antiretroviral medications have been shown to both prolong life and improve the quality of life in people infected with HIV. Although the side effects of antiretroviral medications can be significant, the benefits associated with their use, for example, slowed disease progression and a decrease in HIV-related events, usually outweigh their burdens. However, the benefit/burden balance shifts when patients enter the terminal stages of AIDS. Then, the adverse side effects of antiretroviral medications, for example, nausea, neuropathy, and diarrhea, become more pronounced as the patient's condition deteriorates, thus worsening the patient's quality of life. In addition, no objective evidence supports improvement in a patient's clinical condition when antiretroviral medications are used in the terminal stages of illness.

Because the benefits of antiretroviral medications in the terminal stages of illness are minimal or nonexistent and the disadvantages in terms of untoward effects, multiple medication administration, and scheduling problems are substantial, antiretroviral medications should be avoided during the terminal stages of HIV disease.

Currently, no universally accepted definition of "end-stage HIV disease" exists. However, consensus is emerging regarding the characteristics of patients whose prognosis is less than six months, if the disease runs its normal course. (The National Hospice Organization has published guidelines for determining prognosis in selected non-cancer diseases, including HIV.) The characteristics of patients with end-stage HIV disease generally include a CD4 cell count <25 cells/ul or a viral load of >100,000 copies/ml with the following: failure of all or most antiretroviral regimens, failure of OI treatment, presence of PCNS lymphoma, progressive multi-focal leukoencephalopathy, metastatic cancer, cryptosporidiosis, visceral KS unresponsive to treatment, persistent MAC bacteremia, advanced HIV dementia, toxoplasmosis, or wasting syndrome.

Because medical knowledge regarding appropriate disease-specific therapy for HIV infection is changing continually, physicians should avoid classifying patients as end-stage unless the patient has been evaluated by a physician experienced in treating HIV. A trial of antiretroviral therapy is advisable for patients with very advanced HIV disease who have not had adequate treatment with antiretrovirals in the past, as they may not have received full benefit from these medications.

Approaching Death and Related Psychosocial and Spiritual Issues

Physicians and other healthcare providers tend to focus on the technical aspects of care when dealing with overwhelming illnesses such as HIV disease. The above guidelines are useful when prescribing appropriate palliative treatments, but establishing honest, caring, compassionate relationships with patients and families is one of the most therapeutic interventions a physician can offer.

After palliative care plans have been developed, physicians and other healthcare providers should concentrate on spending time with patients. Taking time to talk with patients about their lives, current or past relationships, and other concerns is not just polite; it provides a powerful opportunity for patients to come to terms with unresolved issues, to explore sources of meaning in their lives, and to achieve a sense of reconciliation and healing.

Because infection with HIV often is acquired through illicit drug use, homosexual activity, or non-monogamous sex, people who are HIV positive commonly experience a sense of shame, which is further exacerbated by the societal stigma associated with an HIV diagnosis. In addition to widespread social stigmatization, patients often experience estrangement from their family members, friends, and community, which leads to a sense of increased isolation just when social support is crucial. Physicians should recognize the potential for reconciliation between patients and their families and encourage it as part of the healing process.

Spiritual reflection usually occurs during the dying process. Questions about meaning, worth, purpose, value, and hope frequently arise. Discussing these and other spiritual issues can foster a rich and rewarding relationship for both patients and physicians. Often, patients want to reestablish connections with their religious tradition, even after years of separation.

Conclusion

Contemporary hospice care evolved largely in response to the needs of patients with end-stage cancer. The hospice and palliative care needs of patients with HIV disease differ from those of cancer patients because appropriate palliation in patients with HIV disease often includes standard disease-specific treatments. This paradigm shift in palliative care has been difficult for some hospice administrators and insurers to appreciate for two reasons: first, they lack understanding of the different needs of patients with HIV disease; and second, reimbursement mechanisms are often inadequate for treatments that provide the best palliation for patients with end-stage HIV disease.

Many communities cope with constraints on hospice care for patients with HIV disease by relying on home health services and avoiding hospice referrals until patients are close to death. This approach is problematic because hospice staff, who are best equipped to help patients and families through the entire terminal phase of illness, are not involved until the final days of a patient's life. Similarly, home health staff, who have developed a relationship with the patient and family, are not involved during the final weeks or days of the patient's life. Reimbursement mechanisms for patients with advanced HIV disease should be evaluated and redesigned so appropriate palliative care is provided by those best trained and equipped to do so.

The hospice and palliative care needs of patients with HIV differ from those of patients with cancer or other systemic diseases. While disease-specific treatments often provide the best palliative therapies for patients with end-stage HIV disease, current reimbursement mechanisms may be inadequate. Physicians and other healthcare providers should take a patient-centered approach to care, provide the best palliative care technically available, and educate others about the special palliative needs of patients with HIV.

Objectives

Attitudes/Behaviors

1. Describe the burdens associated with certain palliative and disease-specific therapies for patients with HIV disease.

2. Describe the need to design palliative regimens that respect a patient's wishes, needs, and ability to tolerate treatment.

3. Discuss when medications used to treat and prevent OIs *and* cancer chemotherapeutic agents are appropriate palliative therapies for patients with end-stage HIV disease.

4. Discuss the burdens and benefits of using antiretroviral therapy in patients with end-stage HIV disease.

5. Describe how the palliative needs of patients with HIV disease differ from those of patients with cancer and other systemic diseases.

6. Discuss the social stigma associated with a diagnosis of HIV disease.

7. Discuss issues of prognostication in patients with HIV disease.

8. Discuss the role of hospice care for patients with end-stage HIV disease.

Knowledge

1. Describe several clinical attributes of end-stage HIV disease.

2. Discuss social, psychological, and spiritual issues often associated with end-stage HIV disease.

3. Describe cost issues related to palliative care for patients with HIV disease.

4. Describe criteria for judging the efficacy of palliative therapies.

5. Describe the treatment and prophylaxis of pneumocystis carinii pneumonia.

6. Discuss the major symptoms associated with cryptococcal meningitis.

7. Describe treatment options for CMV retinitis.

8. Discuss the side effects of treatment for mycobacterium avium complex.

9. Discuss the role of radiation therapy and chemotherapy in the treatment of Kaposi's sarcoma.

10. Describe common symptoms and their treatments in patients with advanced HIV disease.

11. Discuss the common causes of neuropathic pain in patients with HIV disease.

Skills

1. Assess a patient with advanced HIV disease who is using multiple medications, with the goal of adjusting the medications to maximize palliative efficacy.

2. Treat common symptoms in patients with HIV disease.

3. Utilize disease-specific therapy as well as standard palliative therapies when treating a patient with advanced HIV disease.

4. Assess the prognosis of a patient with advanced HIV disease.

5. Recommend appropriate discontinuation of antiretroviral medication in a patient with advanced HIV disease.

6. Work with an interdisciplinary team to manage the multiple contributors to suffering in patients with advanced HIV disease.

References

1. Brettle R, Gore S. Outpatient medical care of injection drug use related HIV. *Int J STD AIDS.* 1992;2(3):96-100.
2. Centers for Disease Control and Prevention. USPHS/IDSA guidelines for the prevention of opportunistic infections in persons infected with HIV: a summary. *MMWR.* 1995;44(RR-8):1-34.
3. Chesney M, et al. Psychological impact of HIV disease and implications for intervention. *Psychiatr Clin North Am.* 1994;17(1):163-82.
4. Deangelis L. Current management of primary central nervous system lymphoma. *Oncology.* 1995; 9(1):63-71.
5. Doyle M, Johnstone P. Role of radiation therapy in management of pulmonary Kaposi's sarcoma. *South Med J.* 1993;86(3):285-8.
6. Foley F, Flannery J. AIDS palliative care- challenging the palliative paradigm. *J Palliat Care.* 1995;11(2):19-22.
7. Folkman S, et al. Stress and coping in caregiving partners of men with AIDS. *Psychiatr Clin North Am.* 1994;17(1):35-53.
8. Forsyth P, Yahalom J. Combined-modality therapy in the treatment of primary central nervous system lymphoma in AIDS. *Neurology.* 1994;44(8):1473-9.
9. Gelmann E, Longo D. Combination chemotherapy of disseminated Kaposi's sarcoma in patients with AIDS. *Am J Med.* 1987;82(3):456-62.
10. Gill P, et al. The effects of preparations of human chorionic gonadotropin on AIDS-related Kaposi's sarcoma. *N Engl J Med.* 1996;335(17):261-9.
11. Hamel R, Lysaught T. Choosing palliative care: do religious beliefs make a difference? *J Palliat Care.* 1994;10(3):61-6.
12. James N, Coker R. Liposomal doxorubicin (Doxil): an effective new treatment for Kaposi's sarcoma in AIDS. *Clin Oncol.* 1994;6(5):294-6.
13. Krook A, Kastrup A. Somatic care wanted by HIV-infected intravenous drug abusers: the patients' opinions and experiences. *AIDS Care.* 1995;7(3):375-79.
14. Lazzarini Z, Reiter G. Integrating legal options for guardianship and adoption into comprehensive HIV related social services. *Proceedings HIV Infection in Women.* 1995;S64.
15. Mattison A, et al. Lesbians, gay men and their families. *Psychiatr Clin North Am.* 1994;17(1):123-37.
16. O'Connor PG, Selwyn PA, Schottenfeld RS. Medical care for injection-drug users with human immunodeficiency virus infection. *New Engl J Med.* 1994;331:450-457.

17. Raju P, Roy T. Palliative radiation therapy for Kaposi's sarcoma in patients with AIDS. *Mo Med.* 1990;87(1):26-8.
18. Reiter G, Kudler N. HIV and palliative care part I. *AIDS Clin Care.* 1996;8(3):21-6.
19. Reiter G, Kudler N. HIV and palliative care part II. *AIDS Clin Care.* 1996; 8(4):27-34.
20. Reiter G. Beyond DNR. *Am J Hospice Palliat Care.* 1995 November/December; 12(6):34-7.
21. Schmitt FA, et al. Neuropsychological outcome of AZT treatment of patients with AIDS and AIDS related complex. *N Engl J Med.* 1988;319:1573-8.
22. Selik R, Chu S. Trends in infectious diseases and cancers among persons dying of HIV infection in the United States from 1987 to 1992. *Ann Intern Med.* 1995;123:933-6.
23. Standards and Accreditation Committee, Medical Guidelines Task Force. *Medical Guidelines for Determining Prognosis in Selected Non-Cancer Diseases*, 2nd ed. Arlington, Va: National Hospice Organization; 1996.
24. Treisman G, et al. Psychiatric care for patients with HIV infection. *Psychosomatics.* 1993; 34(5):433-9.
25. Von Gunten C, Martinez J. AIDS and hospice. *Am J Hospice Palliat Care.* 1991; 4:17-9.
26. Von Gunten C, Martinez J. AIDS and palliative medicine: medical treatment issues. *J Palliat Care.* 1995;11(2):5-9.
27. Zegans L, et al. Psychotherapies for the person with HIV disease. *Psychiatr Clin North Am.* 1994;17(1):149-62.

Hospice and Palliative Medicine for Patients with Non-Cancer Illnesses

Access to Hospice Care for Non-Cancer Patients

In the United States, hospice care developed in response to a need for comprehensive care for terminally ill patients, with emphasis on effective management of pain and other symptoms. In the past, the overwhelming majority of hospice patients had cancer diagnoses; however, during the 1980s, hospice and palliative care programs expanded their services to meet the needs of patients with diagnoses other than cancer. By 1994, 40 percent of hospice patients in the United States had primary diagnoses other than cancer—almost 10 percent had heart disease, predominately congestive heart failure (CHF).

As the incidence of chronic disease increases, patients with non-cancer diseases are likely to represent a higher percentage of hospice and palliative care patients, particularly in view of the need for more cost-effective approaches for managing the end stages of chronic diseases, such as advanced CHF. Because the needs of patients with non-cancer diseases can be as great as, if not greater than, those with cancer, hospice and palliative care services should be available for all terminally ill patients, regardless of diagnosis.

The Dilemma of Prognosis in Non-Cancer Disease

Difficulties predicting prognosis contribute to physician reluctance to refer patients for hospice care. When physicians cannot reliably prognosticate length of life, they are unlikely to certify a patient as eligible for the Medicare Hospice Benefit (MHB), which requires a life expectancy of six months or less, if the disease runs it normal course. Data from the SUPPORT study documented serious shortcomings in end-of-life care for hospitalized patients in the United States, and indicated difficulties with prognosis in inpatients with advanced disease. Just one week prior to a patient's death, attending physicians incorrectly estimated that the median SUPPORT patient had a 50 percent chance of living two months. On the day prior to a patient's death, the median patient was given about a 17 percent chance of living for two months, and a 7 percent chance of living for six months.

The prognostic challenges associated with cancer become even more problematic with advanced non-cancer diseases, such as heart, lung, and Alzheimer's diseases. Contributors to the prognostic dilemma include the following:

- Typically, non-cancer patients experience periods of relative stability interrupted by sudden and often unpredictable exacerbations and downturns, whereas cancer patients tend to experience a fairly relentless and relatively predictable downhill course;
- Exacerbations of heart or lung disease may be almost completely reversible with treatment even in advanced cases, but exacerbations of advanced cancers rarely respond to treatment;
- Even when their disease is quite advanced, patients with non-cancer diseases may not experience the same degree of anorexia, cachexia, and weakness as cancer patients, who usually look and feel extremely ill when they reach the end stage of their disease;
- Effective palliative interventions may affect outcome, e.g., the clinical condition of some terminally ill patients may plateau and some moribund patients may improve due to hospice interventions, such as symptom control, emotional and spiritual support, and nutritional counseling.

Among patients with non-cancer diseases, those with heart and lung disease have the highest rates of referral for hospice care, although predicting the prognosis of patients with these diseases is even more difficult than usual. For example, patients with chronic obstructive pulmonary disease (COPD) are nearest death when exacerbations of their disease require intubation and mechanical ventilation; however, it is impossible, using data readily available to clinicians, to forecast mortality reliably even in such critically ill patients.

Prognostic dilemmas interfere not only with certifying patients for the MHB, but also with recertifying patients for additional benefit periods or discharging them due to extended prognoses. When a patient's condition improves or plateaus after admission to hospice, clinical judgment should be combined with criteria in the National Hospice Organization's (NHO) *Medical Guidelines for Prognosis in Selected Non-Cancer Diseases* to determine a patient's continued eligibility for hospice care. When recertifying patients for the MHB, consideration should also be given to the risk of rapid deterioration in the patient's condition if hospice services are discontinued. Physician involvement is extremely important when patients are being considered for certification, recertification, discharge due to extended prognosis, and readmission for hospice care.

Issues of Palliative Versus Life-Prolonging Treatments

Unlike cancer, no clear distinction exists between treatments to control symptoms and treatments to prolong life in patients with non-cancer diseases. In some cases, a patient's life may be prolonged as a direct result of successful symptom control. For example, in CHF, as in cancer, morphine can palliate dyspnea but it may also have beneficial effects on venous capacitance, reducing preload and congestive symptoms.

In non-cancer diseases, the cause of death often is directly related to treatable complications instead of the disease process. For example, at least 25 percent of male patients with advanced CHF die, not from pulmonary edema itself, but from ventricular arrhythmias. Patients with end-stage pulmonary disease routinely die, not from emphysema, but from sudden pulmonary infections. Because such complications are potentially reversible, physicians usually manage them aggressively unless advance planning documents provide other instructions. To avoid unwanted emergency visits and hospitalizations, physicians and other members of the hospice team must educate patients, family members, and caregivers about treatment decisions, appropriate responses to disease-specific complications the patient is likely to experience, and helpful responses to unexpected and distressing events.

The NHO Medical Guidelines

The NHO developed the *Medical Guidelines for Prognosis in Selected Non-Cancer Diseases* in response to difficulties with prognosis, instances of inappropriate certification of patients for the MHB, and requests from the Health Care Financing Administration (HCFA) for a set of objective criteria to help determine six-month prognosis. The second edition of the *Guidelines* addresses the following diagnostic categories: heart, lung, and Alzheimer's diseases, HIV, liver and renal diseases, stroke/coma, and amyotrophic lateral sclerosis (ALS). NHO distributed the *Guidelines* to every hospice program in the United States, and they are now in widespread use.

Whenever possible, the *Guidelines* were based on scientific studies of mortality in non-cancer disease but they remain a consensus statement that is not yet entirely evidence-based. Eventually, Medicare claims data and other research should help establish the criteria's predictive validity. In addition, statistical methods may be applied to improve their accuracy. Ongoing research is likely to contribute to further negotiations between hospice providers and HCFA for years to come.

Physicians specializing in hospice and palliative medicine should become familiar with the *Guidelines* and stay abreast of revisions as they occur, not only to ensure more accurate prognostication but also to protect the financial health of their hospice programs; that is, reimbursement for hospice services for patients covered by the MHB is contingent on appropriate prognosis.

Summary of Selected NHO Guidelines

The following is a summary of selected sections of the *Guidelines*. For further details and the guidelines for renal disease, stroke/coma, and amyotrophic lateral sclerosis, please obtain a copy of the *Guidelines*.

I. **General Guidelines**: Apply to any candidate for hospice admission. May be used for patients without a formal medical diagnosis.
A. Patient's condition is life-limiting, and patient/family have been informed.
B. Treatment goal is symptom relief rather than cure.
C. Patient has one of the following:
   1. Documented clinical progression of disease or diminished functional status.
   2. Recent impaired nutritional status.

II. **Heart Disease**: A and B should be present.
A. Symptomatic at rest.
   1. New York Heart Association Class IV.
   2. Ejection fraction $\leq 20\%$ (if available).
B. Optimally treated.
   1. Diuretics.
   2. Vasodilators.
C. Other factors.
   1. Refractory arrhythmias.
   2. History of cardiac arrest.
   3. History of syncope.
   4. History of cardiogenic brain embolism.
   5. Progressive HIV disease.

III. **Lung Disease**: A-D should be present.
A. Severe lung disease.
   1. Dyspnea at rest.
   2. Unresponsive to bronchodilators.
   3. Post-bronchodilator $FEV_1 < 30\%$ of predicted (if available).
B. Progressive lung disease.
   1. Recent ER, hospital treatment.
   2. FEV_1 loss of 40 ml in one year (if available).

C. Hypoxemia at rest.
  1. O_2 saturation < 88% on room air, or
  2. P_{O_2} < 55 mm Hg on room air (if available).
D. CO_2 retention (if available): P_{CO_2} > 50 mm Hg.
E. Other factors.
  1. Evidence of cor pulmonale (if available).
  2. Unintentional weight loss of > 10% body weight in 6 months.
  3. Resting heart rate > 100/min.

IV. **Alzheimer's Disease:** A and B should be present.
A. Severe dementia: All of the following; #1 is critical.
  1. Cannot ambulate independently.
  2. Unable to use > 6 different words in meaningful conversation.
  3. Urinary and fecal incontinence.
  4. Unable to dress independently.
  5. Unable to bathe independently.
B. Medical complication: At least one of the following within the last year, severe enough to consider treatment whether or not it was actually provided.
  1. Aspiration pneumonia.
  2. Pyelonephritis.
  3. Sepsis.
  4. Decubitus ulcers, stage III-IV.
  5. Fever, recurrent after antibiotics.
  6. Impaired nutrition; includes patients with feeding tube.
    a. Weight loss > 10% in 6 months.
    b. Serum albumin < 2.5 gm/dl.

V. **HIV Disease:** A-C should be present.
A. CD4+ count < 25/mcL, **OR**
B. Viral load > 100,000 copies/ml.
C. Infectious/neoplastic complication, untreated or refractory: At least one of the following.
  1. CNS lymphoma.
  2. Progressive multifocal leukoencephalopathy.
  3. Cryptosporidiosis.
  4. Wasting (loss of > 33% lean body mass).
  5. MAC bacteremia.

  6. Visceral Kaposi's sarcoma.
  7. Renal failure.
  8. Advanced AIDS dementia.
  9. Toxoplasmosis.
D. Other factors.
  1. Diarrhea > 1 year.
  2. Serum albumin < 2.5 gm/dl.
  3. Substance abuse.
  4. Age > 50.
  5. Foregoing antiretroviral and prophylactic therapy.
  6. Congestive heart failure.

V. **Liver Disease:** A and B should be present.
A. Laboratory indicators: Both should be present.
  1. Prothrombin time > 5 sec. over control, or INR > 1.5.
  2. Serum albumin < 2.5 gm/dl.
B. Clinical syndromes: At least one of the following.
  1. Ascites, refractory to sodium restriction and diuretics.
  2. Spontaneous bacterial peritonitis.
  3. Hepatorenal syndrome.
  4. Hepatic encephalopathy, refractory to protein restriction and lactulose.
  5. Recurrent variceal bleeding.
C. Other factors.
  1. Progressive malnutrition.
  2. Muscle wasting.
  3. Active alcoholism.
  4. Hepatocellular carcinoma.
  5. Positive HBsAg.

HCFA and the Medical Guidelines

HCFA, which administers the MHB, has increased its surveillance of hospice programs through focused medical reviews performed by regional fiscal intermediaries. In addition, the Office of the Inspector General is expanding its Operation Restore Trust activities from six states to all fifty. The Office of the Inspector General has made it clear that hospice programs receiving Medicare reimbursement for services provided to non-eligible patients may be forced to refund the payments. HCFA is using the *Guidelines* as the basis for national Medical Review Policy, which is used by fiscal intermediaries to guide decisions about patient appropriateness and hospice reimbursement. Hospice physicians should be familiar with the content and optimal use of the *Guidelines* to stay in regulatory compliance and, more importantly, to make better decisions about prognosis.

Education and the Medical Guidelines

Active participation by the Hospice Medical Director and staff physicians is crucial when educating hospice staff, referring physicians, and the general medical community about the hospice/palliative medicine approach to patients with non-cancer diseases. The *Guidelines* can be used as a tool for:

- Helping physicans make determinations about prognosis and a patient's eligibility for hospice care;

- Helping referral sources identify patients who might be eligible for the MHB, ideally earlier in the course of their illness;
- Educating referring physicians about effective palliative treatments. For example, despite well-publicized studies documenting the efficacy and safety of high doses of angiotensin-converting enzyme (ACE) inhibitors in advanced CHF, many physicians are reluctant to prescribe dosages adequate to palliate symptoms. Because the *Guidelines* recommend optimal doses of ACE inhibitors as a criterion for admission to hospice, hospice staff can educate community physicians about effective use of ACE inhibitors, thus improving patient care;
- Encouraging training of hospice staff to better palliate symptoms. For example, morphine is routinely used to palliate acute pulmonary edema but may be underutilized for palliation of chronic CHF. Hospice staff are unlikely to successfully palliate end-stage CHF unless they are trained to use morphine effectively, manage volume status with diuretics and vasodilators, and monitor electrolytes, blood pressure, and renal function.

Objectives

Attitudes/Behaviors

1. Describe difficulties associated with determining prognosis in patients with non-cancer diseases and optimal ways of coping with prognostic uncertainty in the hospice environment.

2. Explain the importance of teaching hospice and palliative care nursing staff about effective palliative medical interventions for non-cancer diseases.

3. Explain the sometimes competing needs to improve access to hospice/palliative care services and to accurately predict prognosis in patients with non-cancer diseases.

4. Defend the need to discharge non-cancer patients from the MHB when objective evidence of clinical decline cannot be documented.

5. Describe the role of the NHO *Guidelines* when making decisions about certifying and recertifying non-cancer patients for the MHB.

6. Explain the need to provide hospice/palliative care for patients with non-cancer diseases.

7. Defend the need to provide interdisciplinary team care for terminally ill non-cancer patients.

Knowledge

1. Demonstrate adequate basic knowledge of the physiologic and pathologic processes of non-cancer disease, including CHF, COPD, Alzheimer's, HIV, liver, renal, and neurologic disease.

2. Demonstrate competence in basic pharmacology and therapeutics related to non-cancer diseases.

3. Explain medical issues related to prognosis in patients with non-cancer diseases.

4. Describe the current federal regulatory structure, including the Health Care Financing Administration/Fiscal Intermediary relationship, Office of the Inspector General, and Operation Restore Trust.

5. Explain the basic content of NHO *Guidelines* for each diagnostic category.

6. Describe functional status indicators including the Karnofsky Performance Status and Activities of Daily Living.

7. State two parameters of nutritional deficiency that have been shown to correlate with increased mortality in patients with non-cancer diseases.

8. Define "optimal treatment" for patients with advanced CHF.

9. List three criteria that might help qualify a COPD patient for coverage by the MHB.

10. Describe two critical disabilities related to dementia that may qualify a patient for coverage by the MHB.

11. List two medical complications that help qualify a patient with either Alzheimer's disease or the chronic phase of stroke for coverage by the MHB.

12. State two laboratory tests that are critical for defining terminality in end-stage liver disease.

Skills

1. Determine a non-cancer patient's eligibility for the MHB.

2. Utilize the NHO *Guidelines* when helping nursing staff determine a non-cancer patient's eligibility for continued hospice care under the MHB.

3. Explain to interdisciplinary members, hospice staff, patients, and family members the need to discharge a non-cancer patient from the MHB.

4. Apply current medical knowledge to help the interdisciplinary team develop appropriate treatment plans for patients with non-cancer diseases.

5. Effectively treat distressing symptoms experienced by patients with non-cancer diseases.

6. Demonstrate non-confrontational problem-solving behaviors when discussing a non-cancer patient's eligibility for hospice care with regulatory agencies.

References

1. A controlled trial to improve care for seriously ill hospitalized patients. The study to understand prognoses and preferences for outcomes and risks of treatments (SUPPORT). The SUPPORT Principal Investigators. *JAMA*. 1995;274:1591-8.
2. Bourassa MG, Gurne O, Bangdiwala SI, Ghali JK, et al. For the SOLVD Investigators. Natural history and patterns of current practice in heart failure. *J Am Coll Cardiol*. 1993;22:14A-19A.
3. CONSENSUS Trial Study Group. Effects of enalapril on mortality in severe congestive heart failure: results of the Cooperative North Scandinavian Enalapril Survival Study (CONSENSUS). *N Engl J Med*. 1987;316:1429-35.
4. Christakis N, Escarce J. Survival of Medicare patients after enrollment in hospice programs. *N Engl J Med*. 1996;335:172-8.
5. Garg R, Packer M, Pitt B, Yusuf S. Heart failure in the 1990s: evolution of a major public health problem in cardiovascular medicine. *J Am Coll Cardiol*. 1993;22:3A-5A.
6. Ghali JK, Cooper R, Ford EF. Trends in hospitalization rates for heart failure in the United States, 1973-1986: evidenced for increasing population prevalence. *Arch Intern Med*. 1990;150:769-73.
7. Haupt BJ. Characteristics of patients receiving hospice care services: United States, 1994. *Advance Data*, No. 282. Hyattsville, Md: National Center for Health Statistics; March 6, 1997.
8. Kaelin RM, et al. Failure to predict six month survival of patients with COPD requiring mechanical ventilation by analysis of simple indices: a prospective study. *Chest*. 1987;92:971-8.
9. Lynn, J. An 88-year old woman facing the end of life. *JAMA*. 1997;277(20):1633-1640.
10. Lynn J, Harrell F, Cohn F, Wagner D, Connors AF. Prognoses of seriously ill hospitalized patients on the days before death: implications for patient care and public policy. *New Horiz*. 1997;5(1): 56-61.
11. O'Connell JB and Bristow MR. Economic impact of heart failure in the United States: time for a different approach. *J Heart Lung Transplant*. 1993;13:S107-12.
12. Stuart B, Alexander C, Arenella C, Connor S, et al. Standards and Accreditation Committee, Medical Guidelines Task Force, National Hospice Organization. *Medical Guidelines for Determining Prognosis in Selected Non-Cancer Diseases*, 2nd ed. *Hospice J*. 1996;11:47-63.
13. SOLVD Investigators. Effect of enalapril on survival in patients with reduced left ventricular ejection fractions and congestive heart failure. *N Engl J Med*. 1991;325:293-302.

Psychosocial Aspects of Hospice and Palliative Medicine

Most physicians enthusiastically endorse the concept of comprehensive, whole-person care as a desirable goal, if not an essential component, of excellent patient care. In practice, however, the psychosocial aspects of patient care often are viewed by physicians with dread, bewilderment, or disdain.

Attending to the psychosocial issues experienced by patients with life-limiting illnesses is a crucial component of excellent palliative medicine. No other area of medical practice requires more mastery of the art of medicine, more gentle attention to bedside manner, and more empathic participation in the doctor-patient relationship than caring for seriously ill patients and their family members. Rarely do patients in any other phase of the life cycle need as much assistance with the psychosocial aspects of their illness as do patients nearing the end of life.

During the latter phases of life, patients often experience psychosocial problems, such as interpersonal or family conflict, marital discord, occupational and financial problems, spiritual and existential distress, and psychological and emotional distress unrelated to a formal mental disorder. However, patients may not relate their concerns without gentle prompting from the physician.

With the patient's approval, physicians can and should share many of the patient's psychosocial problems with other members of the treatment team (or refer such problems to other team members altogether), but hospice and palliative medicine physicians should also know how to elicit, identify, and respond to such issues. Even when interventions for a problem do not include medical interventions, acknowledgment by the doctor that such problems are important and worthy of attention is, by itself, healing.

Skillful management of psychosocial issues requires attention to potential causes of suffering, acknowledgment of the patient's and family's grief, the provision of caring support, consideration of the patient's subjective quality of life, and ongoing bereavement support. Addressing a patient's psychosocial issues provides palliative care professionals with important opportunities to guide and support patients and families in their search for a renewed sense of hope, meaning, and continued personal growth.

Suffering

American medical training emphasizes the diagnosis of distinct disease states, the application of tested therapies, and the prognostication of outcomes. This approach is referred to as the medical-biological model of care and has proved to be a powerful and versatile tool for generations of physicians. However, not all causes of patient distress fit easily into a disease construct; some are better addressed by a more empathic, narrative approach to care.

Cassell's concept of suffering provides a more comprehensive and helpful framework for understanding a patient's distress. He suggests that, although symptoms arise from clinical disease states, suffering is experienced by persons. Physical symptoms such as pain, nausea, constipation, and dyspnea can be major causes of suffering, but so can non-physical symptoms such as depression and anxiety. According to Cassell, suffering can occur in relation to any aspect of personhood. He summarizes suffering in this way: *Suffering occurs when an impending destruction of the person is perceived; it continues until the threat of disintegration has passed or until the integrity of the person can be restored in some other manner.*

Contributors to Suffering

Beliefs

Beliefs about the meaning of illness and health can cause suffering among patients and families. Patients with illnesses that are stigmatizing or otherwise dreaded in the patient's culture (e.g., AIDS, cancer) may suffer as a consequence of the perceived meaning of their illness. Illnesses with lifestyle-related risk factors can cause distressing feelings of guilt and shame. Concerns about contagion, even if irrational, can also cause great distress for patients and families. Symptoms such as pain may be interpreted by patients as terrible signs that the disease is progressing rapidly toward death, or the symptoms may be tolerated with pride as a badge of courage. Styles of coping can also contribute to suffering, particularly if the patient does not possess adequate coping skills for adapting to the stresses and challenges of a terminal illness.

Past experiences

Past experiences with illness may contribute to suffering, particularly when patients suffer from recurrent illnesses and can recall suffering associated with previous episodes of the disease. The experiences of friends and family members with the same or similar illnesses also can be significant contributors to suffering, particularly if their distress was inadequately controlled.

Conflict

Interpersonal conflict, particularly among family members, adds greatly to the burden of suffering in terminal illness. Other types of conflict, including the following, also contribute to suffering: care system conflicts (e.g., disagreements among care providers about proposed treatments, poor coordination of care, etc.); interpersonal conflicts with physicians; communication problems with other members of the care team; and financial conflicts due to health care expenses. Resolution of conflicts, when possible, not only lessens the patient's suffering but also lightens the load for family members, who must grieve the loss of a loved one.

Role function

The debilitating impact of an illness on a patient's ability to perform significant roles (e.g., spouse or partner, parent, child, employee, friend, or citizen) also contributes to suffering. To help physicians understand the psychosocial implications of an illness, they should consider its impact on the patient's ability to perform meaningful roles.

Impairment

Impairments in the functional domain also contribute to suffering, for example, physical impairments caused by the illness, physical complications of the illness, and diminished strength due to limited activity.

Culture

Patients with advanced illnesses exist and suffer within the context of their culture. In addition to the patient's personal historical context, particular cultural and historical contexts must also be considered. The patient's family, extended social system, and community often provide support and relief of suffering, but they can also be sources of additional suffering. Other cultural contexts that influence suffering near the end of life include isolation from culture-specific sources of social support, regional variations in culture, the patient's national or ethnic culture, and the patient's own religious and spiritual beliefs.

Spiritual and existential concerns

Spiritual and existential concerns may add to suffering. A diagnosis of terminal illness typically forces patients to reconsider sources of meaning in their lives. Plans for the future must be reviewed and revised, and some plans must be abandoned, which contributes to suffering. Regrets and misgivings about the past may cause a great deal of suffering. Patients may believe that their illness is a form of punishment for past deeds. They may be concerned about life after death or the welfare of loved ones who will be left behind.

Loss of independence and control

Loss of independence and control can be sources of suffering for patients, particularly for those with high control needs. Distress associated with lack of control over bodily functions and impaired psychological and cognitive functioning also cause suffering. These changes can be as painful for family members to witness as they are for the patient to endure.

Sexuality and intimacy

Issues related to sexuality and intimacy often are ignored by healthcare professionals and family members. Healthcare professionals should specifically inquire about the sexual and intimacy concerns of patients and their significant others. Some patients and their significant others desire ongoing expressions of sexuality and intimacy. Others, who may have avoided physical or emotional intimacy during their relationship, may be deeply fearful of expectations about providing personal care or discussing personal issues.

For patients with advanced disease, expressions of sexuality often involve more than the act of intercourse—they can include cuddling, caressing, and other physical expressions of warmth and caring. Physical manifestations of intimacy can include helping with personal care, grooming, and appearance.

Interventions

All of the above sources of suffering, as well as others not listed, can and should be addressed if they are detected. Effective interventions, though not medical in the strictest sense, can be of great benefit to patients and family members. Often, suffering can be alleviated before formal interventions are initiated just by the simple act of listening to the patient's story, exploring causes of suffering, and helping the patient construct a renewed sense of meaning.

The therapeutic benefits of life review are substantial. Encouraging patients to tell stories about their lives and helping them identify positive themes in those stories, such as raising a family, contributing their time to subjectively important causes, enduring hardships, and so on, can help patients discover a renewed sense of meaning, self-worth, and value in their lives.

Assistance with achieving specific goals can also be a great source of comfort near the end of life, for example, facilitating attendance at meaningful family events, assisting with the completion of a cherished project, or helping with the resolution of unfinished business.

Grief and Bereavement

Parkes defines bereavement as "the situation of anyone who has lost a person to whom they are attached." Grief is defined as the psychological and emotional reactions to bereavement. Mourning is the social face of grief. Grief can occur in reaction to an actual loss or in anticipation of a loss, that is, anticipatory grief. Grief and bereavement are experienced by dying patients, family members, friends, and medical caregivers. A wide range of normal grief reactions exists— individual variation is the rule, not the exception. When complicated or pathological grief occurs, immediate therapeutic attention is important.

Various "stages of grief" have been proposed. They are interesting from a historical perspective and can be helpful for understanding grief as a process, but they should not be viewed as universal frameworks for grieving. Rigid adherence to theoretical systems of grief ignores individual variations among grieving people, cultures, and communities. Individuals often vacillate between so-called stages of grief, experience phases simultaneously or out of sequence, or skip stages altogether.

Common symptoms of grief, especially in the acute stage, may be incorrectly interpreted as pathologic. Tearfulness, emotional numbness, waves of acute grief, searching for the lost person, feelings of unreality about the death, and brief nondelusional hallucinations of the deceased are all normal physical, psychological, and emotional reactions to bereavement. No reliable rules about "normal" time frames for grief exist, but acute reactions to bereavement generally lessen and resolve over time—usually in terms of months or years rather than days or weeks.

Complicated bereavement may be indicated if the grieving process is avoided, inhibited, delayed, conflicted, or chronic. Self-loathing or suicidal ideation are not components of the normal grieving process. Grief can be complicated by psychiatric disorders such as major depression, panic disorder, or alcohol dependence. Such comorbid problems add greatly to suffering and should be treated aggressively. Bereavement and grief may also have adverse effects on the physical health of the grieving person, ranging from increases in risky health behaviors to increases in mortality after a loss.

Cultural and religious differences affect not only the response and adaptation to loss but also the rituals associated with death and funerals. Grief responses differ according to gender, coping style, access to social support, the health status of the grieving person, and age, which is particularly important to remember when dealing with children. A child's understanding of loss and his/her response to bereavement are strongly influenced by

developmental stages, cognitive and emotional development, and personal experiences.

Interventions to assist with the bereavement process should begin before the patient's death. Overall, the focus of care should be on the whole family, not just on the patient. Excellent symptom control, diligent patient and family education, and ready availability of emotional support can ease the family's burden when caring for a dying relative. If indicated, efforts should be made to resolve interpersonal conflicts. Helping family members understand the important but often enigmatic communications of dying patients ("final gifts"), can also comfort the family.

Interventions to assist with the process of grieving vary, often depending on whether a grieving person is screened and receives services proactively, or is treated only after a referral is made. Though few physicians personally provide specialized bereavement care, they should be able to offer basic interventions, which are almost universally helpful. In addition to providing excellent palliative care before the patient's death, physicians should offer to meet with the family after the patient's death to provide support and to answer questions. When complicated bereavement occurs, physicians should make referrals to professionals specializing in grief and bereavement counseling.

Quality of Life

When cure is no longer a reasonable expectation, optimizing the patient's quality of life becomes the main concern. Quality of life (QOL) is measured by a subjective assessment of the degree to which a patient's perceived essential needs are being met. Poor quality of life is closely related to suffering, which can be understood as the distress experienced by a patient whose essential needs are not being met.

Assessing contributors to a patient's suffering is an important first step in alleviating distress and helping patients maximize the quality of their remaining life. By listening carefully to a patient's story and identifying and providing interventions for specific physical, social, emotional, and spiritual contributors to suffering, healthcare professionals can help patients and families regain a sense of hope and worth and begin to realize that life can be profoundly meaningful, even near the end of life.

Formal instruments for measuring QOL are used most frequently in research settings. Such instruments have limited application in the clinical setting, but they can be helpful in some situations. Some QOL instruments lack the brevity needed for use with profoundly ill patients, and others focus too narrowly on specific contributors to quality of life, such as physical impairment or role functioning. Ideally, instruments measuring QOL in the clinical setting should take into account the subjective nature of suffering and quality of life. It is important to remember that individuals vary significantly in the value they place on specific health and QOL factors, not only throughout their life span but also as their disease progresses. Though quantitative measures of quality of life are frequently desirable, no currently available instrument can replace careful empathic interviewing as a means of ascertaining a patient's values, priorities, and perceptions of quality of life.

Objectives

Attitudes/Behaviors

1. Demonstrate understanding and belief in the importance of attending to psychosocial aspects of palliative care.

2. Demonstrate understanding and belief in the value of simultaneous evaluation and treatment using the biological-medical approach and the empathic-narrative approach.

3. Display concern for and willingness to initiate evaluation of suffering and quality of life in the dying patients and their family members.

4. Display concern for grieving and bereaved individuals and demonstrate a willingness to intervene.

5. Demonstrate a willingness and ability to refer grieving persons to other caregivers when appropriate.

6. Demonstrate understanding of differences in cultural approaches to death and dying.

7. Describe the individual variation in the normal response to bereavement.

8. Describe the importance of preserving subjectivity in assessing quality of life.

9. Discuss the importance of life review when caring for a patient with advanced disease.

10. Describe the importance of inquiring about sexuality and intimacy when caring for a patient with advanced disease.

11. Defend the concept that patients with advanced disease can experience a sense of hope, worth, and meaning near the end of life.

Knowledge

1. Describe the multifaceted responsibilities of the physician when caring for the patient with advanced incurable disease.

2. Define grief, mourning, bereavement, anticipatory grief, and pathological grief.

3. Outline a general approach to evaluation of suffering in the dying patient and describe major sources of suffering.

4. List several sources of impaired quality of life for patients near the end of life.

5. Outline a general approach to evaluation of grief and bereavement in the dying patient and his or her family.

6. Summarize the concepts of stages of grief.

7. List several factors which commonly complicate grief.

8. List adverse outcomes of prolonged or complicated grief.

9. Recognize the common symptoms and manifestations of grief.

10. Cite at least five symptoms of unresolved grief.

11. Summarize theories of the tasks of grief and bereavement.

12. Describe variables which may influence normal grief, including the grieving person's gender, cultural background, religious tradition, age, coping style, health, access to social support, and personal experiences.

13. Define quality of life.

14. Describe an approach to clinical assessment of quality of life.

15. Describe the features of an ideal quality-of-life assessment instrument.

Skills

1. Assess suffering in patients near the end of life.

2. Outline a management plan for multiple causes of suffering.

3. Balance biological and psychosocial factors in assessment and management of suffering in the patient near the end of life.

4. Describe at least five ways to lessen the burden of suffering for patients and families in the last days of life.

5. Develop a management plan for normal or abnormal grief.

6. Differentiate between grief problems likely to respond to simple interventions and grief problems that may need specialized attention.

7. Identify quality of life problems in individual patients.

8. Demonstrate a working understanding of clinical quality-of-life assessment.

9. Demonstrate the ability to address the typical fears and emotional reactions dying patients experience.

10. Demonstrate a working understanding of the most frequently used quality-of-life assessment instruments.

References

1. Aaronson NK, Ahmedzai S, Bergman B, et al. The European Organization for Research and Treatment of Cancer QLQ-C30: a quality-of-life instrument for use in international clinical trials in oncology. *J Natl Cancer Inst.* 1993;85:365-376.
2. Callanan M, Kelley P. *Final Gifts: Understanding the Special Awareness, Needs, and Communications of the Dying.* New York: Simon and Schuster; 1992.
3. Cassell EJ. The nature of suffering. *New Eng J Med.* 1982;306:639-645.
4. Cassell EJ: *The Nature of Suffering and the Goals of Medicine.* New York: Oxford University Press; 1991.
5. Cassem NH: The dying patient. In: Cassem NH, ed. *Massachusetts General Hospital Handbook of General Hospital Psychiatry*, 3rd ed. St. Louis: Mosby Year Book; 1991:343-371.
6. Cella DF, Tulsky DS, Gray G, et al. The Functional Assessment of Cancer Therapy Scale: development and validation of the general measure. *J Clin Oncol.* 1993;11:570-579.
7. Cherny NI, Coyle N, Foley KM. Suffering in the advanced cancer patient: a definition and taxonomy. *J Palliat Care.* 1994;10:57-70.
8. Corr CA, Doka KJ. Current models of death, dying, and bereavement. *Crit Care Nurs Clin North Am.* 1994;6:545-552.
9. Gregory D, English JC. The myth of control: suffering in palliative care. *J Palliat Care.* 1994;10(2):18-22.
10. Hull MM. Hospice nurses. Caring support for caregiving families. *Cancer Nurs.* 1991; 14(2):63-70.
11. Irish DP, Lundquist KF, Nelsen VJ. *Ethnic Variations in Dying, Death, and Grief.* Washington, DC: Taylor and Francis; 1993.
12. Jacobsen PB, Breitbart W. Psychosocial aspects of palliative care. *Cancer Control.* 1996;3:214-222.
13. Kornblith AB, Holland JC. *Handbook of Measures for Psychological, Social, and Physical Function in Cancer, Volume I: Quality of Life.* New York: Memorial Sloan-Kettering Cancer Center; 1994.
14. Lamerton R. *Care of the Dying.* New York: Viking Penguin; 1991.
15. Larson DG. *The Helper's Journey, Working With People Facing Grief, Loss, and Life-threatening Illness.* Champaign Ill: Research Press; 1993.
16. McMillan SC, Mahon M. Measuring quality of life in hospice patients using a newly developed Hospice Quality of Life Index. *Qual Life Res.* 1994;3:437-447.
17. Overbeck B, Overbeck J. *What to Do When Someone Dies.* Dallas, Tex: TLC Group;1992.
18. Parkes CM. Bereavement. In: Doyle D, Hanks GWC, MacDonald N, eds. *Oxford Textbook of Palliative Medicine.* Oxford: Oxford University Press; 1993:665-678.
19. *Pathways for Facing Terminal Illness.* Arlington, Va: National Hospice Organization; 1997.
20. Rando TA. *Grief, Dying, and Death.* Champaign, Ill: Research Press Company; 1984.
21. Rando TA. *Treatment of Complicated Mourning.* Champaign, Ill: Research Press Company; 1993.
22. Saunders CM, ed. *The Management of Terminal Disease.* New York: Williams and Wilkins; 1985.
23. Schipper H, Clinch J, Murray A, et al. Measuring the quality of life of cancer patients: the Functional Living Index—cancer: development and validation. *J Clin Oncol.* 1984;2:472-483.
24. Shuster JL, Jones GR. Approach to the patient receiving palliative care. In: Stern TA, Herman J, eds. *Practical Guide to Psychiatry for Primary Care Clinicians.* Boston, Mass: Little, Brown and Co: 1998.
25. Slevin ML. Who should measure quality of life, the doctor or the patient? *Br J Cancer.* 1988; 57:109-112.
26. Vachon MLS, Kristjanson L, Higginson I. Psychosocial issues in palliative care: the patient, the family, and the process and outcome of care. *J Pain Symptom Manage.* 1995;10:142-150.
27. Verhulst J. The role of the psychiatrist: defining methods, theories, and practice in the time of managed care. *Acad Psychiatr.* 1996; 20:195-204.

28. Viney L, Walker BM, Robertson T, et al. Dying in palliative care units and in hospital: a comparison of the quality of life of terminal cancer patients. *J Consult Clin Psychol.* 1994; 62:157-164.
29. Warner SC, Wiliams JI. The Meaning in Life Scale: determining the reliability and validity of a measure. *J Chron Dis.* 1987;40:503-12.
30. Watson MA. Bereavement in the elderly. *AORN J.* 1994;59(5):1079-1084.
31. Weissman AD, Hackett TP. Predilection to death: death and dying as a psychiatric problem. *Psychosom Med.* 1961;23:232-256.
32. Worden JW. *Grief Counseling and Grief Therapy,* 2nd ed. New York: Springer Pub Co; 1991.
33. Yates JW, Chalmer B, McKegney FP. Evaluation of patients with advanced cancer using the Karnofsky Performance Status. *Cancer.* 1980;45:2220-2224.
34. Zisook S, Schneider D, Shuchter SR. Anxiety and bereavement. *Psychiatr Med.* 1990;8:83-96.
35. Zisook S, Shuchter SR. Uncomplicated bereavement. *J Clin Psychiatry.* 1993;54:365-72.
36. Zisook S, Shuchter SR, Sledge PA, et al. The spectrum of depressive phenomena after spousal bereavement. *J Clin Psychiatry.* 1994;55:29-36. (suppl)

MODULE SEVENTEEN

Spiritual Aspects of Hospice and Palliative Medicine

Multidimensional Nature of Suffering

When caring for patients with life-threatening illnesses, physicians quickly discover the multidimensional nature of suffering and begin to appreciate the need for interventions beyond those associated with the biomedical model of medicine. See Module Sixteen for a definition of suffering and a discussion of its psychosocial aspects.

Over the past two decades, remarkable progress has been made in treating the physical dimensions of suffering, but no universally recognized interventions exist for treating the spiritual or transcendent dimensions. In fact, no commonly accepted definitions of spirit or spirituality exist, though most would agree that they differ from religion. Religions are based on a body of theological belief and a relationship within a community of faith. Spirituality and the spirit, like the body and mind, are integral components of human existence; however, like love, their existence cannot be proven, only experienced.

By necessity, explorations of spiritual issues are indirect and occur within the realm of meaning. Currently, no interventions exist which are universally accepted as effective for alleviating spiritual pain. Reliable instruments for measuring the effectiveness of specific spiritual interventions have not yet been developed.

Spiritual suffering, which generally involves a sense of lost meaning, hope, and wholeness, is experienced to some degree by nearly every person approaching the end of life. Due to the intimacy of the therapeutic relationship that often develops between a dying patient and his/her physician, patients and family members may present spiritual issues or concerns that require immediate, skilled attention. In those moments, physicians are called upon to respond with sensitivity, and to serve, however reluctantly, in a "priestly" capacity.

Indicators of Spiritual Suffering

Cassell eloquently distinguishes pain and suffering—the body experiences pain but the entire person experiences suffering. Cassell also suggests that persons consist of many dimensions (e.g., physical, emotional, spiritual, social), each of which is subject to real or perceived losses that can cause suffering. Kearney describes several factors which indicate the likely presence of spiritual suffering, or soul pain:

- Patients and/or family members use words like "anguished" or "tortured" to describe their condition;
- Physical symptoms that normally respond to medical interventions are resistant to therapy;

- Patients experience a sense of agitated struggling, extreme denial, or an all-pervading sense of meaninglessness;
- Patients and/or family members ask existential questions, e.g., "Why me? Why now? What did I do to deserve this?"
- Anger is directed at God, medical personnel who are unable to cure the disease, or the disease itself;
- Patients and/or family members feel a deep sense of guilt or shame about specific past actions which they now regret, or they feel guilty because they believe their actions or beliefs caused the illness;
- Patients feel unfairness or a sense of being let down by God, which can be particularly painful for patients who considered themselves to be religious people and now feel as if they have lost their faith.

NOTE—Existential questions usually begin with "why" and often serve as clues that patients need to explore the deeper meanings of life, not just listen as the physician supplies more information.

The Physician's Role in Addressing Spiritual Issues

In his presentation, *Beyond Physical and Psychosocial Care*, Dr. Balfour Mount asks the question, "Why should I be involved in pastoral care?" when it may have nothing to do with a physician's training or interests. Many factors support the need for physician involvement in spiritual care, including the following:

- Spiritual suffering is nearly ubiquitous in patients with life-threatening illness; physicians can choose to intervene skillfully or poorly. The ability to respond to spiritual pain with skill and sensitivity is a crucial component of hospice and palliative medicine.

- The spiritual dimension is relational; whenever physicians interact with profoundly ill patients and their family members, the spiritual dimension is present and cannot be avoided.
- Because the physical and spiritual domains of personhood are interconnected, optimum control of physical symptoms may require the alleviation of spiritual pain. Learning to recognize the complex factors that contribute to suffering increases the physician's ability to intervene more effectively with state-of-the-art medical interventions and with interventions that alleviate spiritual pain.
- A physician's increasing awareness of the full spectrum of a dying patient's needs is likely to result in more effective participation on an interdisciplinary team. Physicans, nurses, chaplains, social workers, and other healthcare professionals must work together to meet the complex interrelated needs of dying patients and their family members. Although each team member represents a specific discipline, each must also respond to the needs of the moment. It is not the sole responsibility of clergy to respond to a patient's spiritual concerns.
- Refusing to respond to a patient's or family member's spiritual concerns closes the door on the possibility of participating in life-enhancing explorations of spiritual issues. When patients trust physicians with deeply felt spiritual concerns, they are likely to be responding to the physician's ability to establish a climate of mutuality, respect, and interdependence, which are essential to the practice of hospice and palliative medicine. When a patient's complex spiritual problems exceed the physician's ability to intervene, the patient should be referred to a specialist in spiritual counseling.
- Some patients and families may not experience spiritual suffering or may not acknowledge its presence. When unacknowledged spiritual issues appear to be contributing to a patient's suffering,

physicians and other team members can provide gentle guidance related to spiritual exploration while respecting the patient's right not to discuss specific problems.

Interventions for Spiritual Healing

- **Listen.** Although the healing power of listening is frequently discounted, when skillfully performed it is a powerful intervention that helps patients reframe painful events and find meaning in their lives. People approach terminal illnesses from multiple perspectives and they frequently have stories they want to tell. Listening to patients as they tell their stories encourages them to review their lives, and helps them find meaning in patterns that emerge. Listening can also provide physicians with important clues about the patient's coping strategies, values, and lifelong concerns. While telling their stories, patients often share important memories, whether pleasant or painful, and describe actions about which they feel proud or ashamed.
- **Explore spiritual issues.** Exploring spiritual issues with patients fosters a deep sense of healing. When patients are suffering from spiritual pain, the process of mutually exploring spiritual issues with empathy and sensitivity is more helpful than trying to provide answers to specific spiritual questions. Most spiritual concerns have no universally accepted answers because they involve questions of worth, value, and meaning.

  Many patients use their spiritual pain to deepen their capacity to love, forgive, and let go. Some patients construct meanings for their illness that help them cope from day to day. Others grow in their understanding and relationship either with God or with the spiritual center of their being—however they may define it. Sometimes, the process of spiritual healing is supported by the patient's close friends, family, and faith community, or by hospice volunteers and healthcare providers who have time to listen. A patient's concerns about the future vary according to past experiences and beliefs.

  - ▶ Typically, patients experience a sense of sustained hope during a terminal illness, although the focus of hope usually changes from hope for a cure to hope for such things as a pain-free death, continued emotional and spiritual support, or future happiness for family members and others who are left behind.

  - ▶ Some patients are fearful about the dying process and seek reassurance about symptom control and continued emotional support for themselves and their family members.

  - ▶ Some patients want to explore concerns about an afterlife. They may use religious or nonreligious frameworks of meaning to explore spiritual issues; both can be beneficial.

- **Help with closure.** It may be important to direct the patient's or family's attention to resolving conflicts, receiving forgiveness, and grieving. When personal and family conflicts can be resolved, it contributes to a peaceful death and eases the bereavement of everyone involved. Patients may appreciate guidance on appropriately channeling anger or reframing events in more helpful ways. Encouraging patients to make a will, discuss funeral arrangements, and complete unfinished emotional and financial business can provide them with valuable strategies for coping with the reality of death.

Growth and Development at the End of Life

Byock suggests that dying is an important identifiable stage in the human life cycle which, like childhood and adolescence, is associated with specific developmental tasks, including the following:

- Completion of worldly affairs
- Completion of relationships with the community
- Completion of relationships with family and friends
- Development of a sense of meaning about life in general and one's life in particular
- Experience of love of self
- Experience of love of others
- Acceptance of the finality of life and of one's existence as an individual
- Development of a sense of self beyond personal loss
- Surrender to the transcendent and the unknown, i.e., letting go of attachments to this world

Clinicians can help patients attain such developmental landmarks by removing impediments (e.g., severe nausea) and by gently suggesting the importance of such tasks when the time is right and the patient is ready to listen. The realization that continued emotional and spiritual growth is possible near the end of life can be profoundly meaningful for patients and families. Assisting patients and families in their search for renewed hope and healing can be one of the most rewarding aspects of hospice and palliative care.

Impact on Physicians

Physicians who care for dying patients frequently discover that the nature of their work leads to confrontations with their own deep feelings about death and personal losses. Unexplored personal feelings of loss and grief can interfere with a physician's ability to intervene effectively when patients are suffering, and may lead to protective ways of relating that discourage patients and family members from sharing spiritual concerns that trouble the physician.

Physicians can benefit professionally and personally by exploring their own feelings of loss and grief. The willingness of health professionals to surrender control over the direction of the spiritual journey and to accompany their patients along the rocky paths of pain, anger, guilt, and grief, sometimes at substantial personal risk, is essential to spiritual care.

Thus, it is important for all health professionals to be aware of the importance of listening to patients and family members and responding to spiritual issues as they arise. Interventions such as listening and exploring spiritual issues can be deeply meaningful not only for patients and families but also for physicians. They help us find meaning and hope, even at the end of life.

Objectives

Attitudes/Behaviors

1. Describe the importance of interventions that support faith, hope, and meaning.

2. Describe spirit as an essential component of personhood and the role of spirit in the contribution to and relief of suffering.

3. Describe the importance of differentiating the physician's spiritual and religious agendas from those of patients and families and explain methods that can be used to avoid imposing the physician's beliefs on the patient.

4. Explain the multidimensional nature of suffering and interventions used by interdisciplinary team members to alleviate suffering in various dimensions of personhood.

5. Describe appropriate and inappropriate uses of denial when employed by physicians—as well as patients and families—in life-threatening therapeutic encounters.

6. Describe a physician's sense of personal helplessness in the face of a patient's terminal illness, and explain how it can be used to improve skills when caring for the dying.

7. Describe the roles of non-medical members of the interdisciplinary team and explain effective strategies for promoting collaboration and respect among various disciplines.

8. Recognize the heterogeneity of religious traditions, beliefs, and practices and explain methods affirming individual experience and avoiding inappropriate generalizations.

9. Describe personal experiences of spiritual suffering and interventions that facilitated healing.

10. Discuss the concept of growth and development near the end of life.

Knowledge

1. Distinguish the common dichotomies encountered in hospice and palliative medicine, such as body and mind, pain and suffering, cure and healing, spirituality and religion.

2. Describe spiritual suffering.

3. Discuss pastoral and religious themes and language and the use of appropriate language when communicating with members of the interdisciplinary team, patients, and families from differing religious traditions.

4. List verbal and nonverbal clues that help distinguish between requests for more medical information and a desire to explore deeper, existential issues.

5. Describe various types of physician/patient relationships and defend those that are likely to encourage the exploration of existential issues.

6. Demonstrate a working knowledge of medical interventions that may increase spiritual suffering in dying patients.

7. Discuss the ethical aspects of spiritual care.

8. Describe various indirect methods, e.g., questionnaires, etc. for revealing unrecognized and/or unresolved spiritual issues.

9. Describe developmental tasks for patients near the end of life

Skills

1. Write or narrate a spiritual autobiography.

2. Identify specific emotional symptoms indicating spiritual distress, e.g., guilt, fear, hopelessness, worthlessness, meaninglessness, etc.

3. Recognize symbolic language indicating spiritual distress, e.g. "tormented," "anguished," "restless," "tortured," etc.

4. Identify patients in spiritual crisis, describe specific interventions that might alleviate their distress, including dream work, meditation, music therapy, etc., and explain why the chosen intervention(s) is appropriate for a specific patient.

5. Obtain a spiritual history.

6. Describe personal techniques for offering professional spiritual support in a non-threatening manner.

7. Facilitate the emotional, spiritual, and philosophical transition of patients and families from hope for survival to transcendental hope.

8. Recognize signs of excellent symptom control and spiritual healing: people become less guilty about the past, less fearful of the future, and more comfortable in the present.

References

1. Ajemian I. The interdisciplinary team. In: Doyle D, Hanks GWC, MacDonald N, eds. *Oxford Textbook of Palliative Medicine*. New York: Oxford University Press; 1993:17-28.
2. Barnard D. The promise of intimacy and the fear of our own undoing. *J Palliat Care*. 1995; 11(9):22-26.
3. Brody H. My story is broken; can you help me fix it? Medical ethics and the joint construction of narrative. *Lit Med*. 1994;13(1):79-92.
4. Byock I. *Dying Well: The Prospect for Growth at the End of Life*. New York: Riverhead Books; 1997.
5. Byock IR. The nature of suffering and the nature of opportunity at the end of life. *Clin Geriatr Med*. 1996;12(2):237-252.
6. Cassell EJ. *The Nature of Suffering and The Goals of Medicine*. New York: Oxford University Press; 1991.
7. Cassell EJ. The importance of understanding suffering for clinical ethics. *J Clin Ethics*. 1991; 2(2):81-82.
8. Davis D. A question of context. *J Clin Ethics*. 1995; Fall:6(3):232-236.
9. Delbanco T. Enriching the doctor-patient relationship by inviting the patient's perspective. *Ann Intern Med*. 1992;116:414-418.
10. Grodin M. Halakhic dilemmas in modern medicine. *J Clin Ethics*. Fall 1995:218-221.
11. Hallenback, J. Cultural considerations of death and dying in America. Presented at the Eighth Annual Assembly of the American Academy of Hospice and Palliative Medicine; June 14, 1996; Snowbird, Utah. Tape available from: Rollin' Recordings, 208 River Ranch Rd, Boerne, Tx, 28006, Tel. 210-537-5494.
12. Herth K. Fostering hope in terminally ill people. *J Adv Nurs*. 1990;15:1250-1259.
13. Kagawa-Singer M. Redefining health: living with cancer. *Soc Sci Med*. 1993;37(2):295-304.
14. Kaplan S, Greenfield S, Gandek B, Rogers W, Ware J. Characteristics of physicians with participatory decision-making styles. *Ann Intern Med*. 1996;124:497-504.
15. Kearney M. *Mortally Wounded*. New York: Scribner; 1996.

16. Kearney M. Spiritual pain. *The Way*. 1991;1(1):47-54.
17. Keller A. Autobiography: finding voice in medical education. Presented at the Annual Meeting of the Society for Health and Human Values; Oct. 26-28, 1989.
18. Lapierre L. A model for describing spirituality. *J Religion Health*. 1994;33(2):153-161.
19. Mandziuk P. Easing chronic pain with spiritual resources. *J Religion Health*. 1993;32(1):47-54.
20. Matthews D, Suchman A, Branch W. What makes the doctor-patient relationship therapeutic? Exploring the connexional dimension of medical care. *Ann Intern Med*. 1988;108:125-30.
21. Muldoon M, King N. Spirituality, health care, and bioethics. *J Religion Health*. 1995;34(4):329-349.
22. Mount, B. Beyond physical and psychosocial care. Presented at the International Hospice Institute Conference; 1990; Estes Park, Colo. (Tape available from: Rollin' Recordings, 208 River Ranch Rd, Boerne, Tx, 28006, Tel. 210-537-5494.)
23. Neuberger J. Cultural issues in palliative care. In: Doyle D, Hanks GWC, MacDonald N, eds. *Oxford Textbook of Palliative Medicine*. New York: Oxford University Press; 1993:505-514.
24. Quill T, Brody H. Physician recommendations and patient autonomy: finding a balance between physician power and patient choice. *Ann Intern Med*. 1996;125:763-769.
25. Rosen I. The spiritual dimension of cognitive therapy. *J Religion Health*. 1991;30(2):93-98.
26. Rosner F. Jewish medical ethics. *J Clin Ethics*. 1995; Fall: 202-217.
27. Schweizer H. To give suffering a language. *Lit Med*. 1995;14(2):210-221.
28. Speck P. Spiritual issues in palliative care. In: Doyle D, Hanks GWC, MacDonald N, eds. *Oxford Textbook of Palliative Medicine*. New York: Oxford University Press; 1993:517-525.
29. Stuart B. Caring for the soul: the deeper mission of hospice and palliative care. Presented at the Eighth Annual Assembly of the American Academy of Hospice and Palliative Medicine; June 13, 1996; Snowbird, Utah. (Tape available from: Rollin' Recordings, 208 River Ranch Rd, Boerne, Tx, 28006, Tel. 210-537-5494)
30. Storey P. The many faces of hope for the terminally ill. Presented at the Eighth Annual Assembly of the American Academy of Hospice and Palliative Medicine; June 13, 1996; Snowbird, Utah. (Tape available from: Rollin' Recordings, 208 River Ranch Rd, Boerne, Tx, 28006, Tel. 210-537-5494)
31. Storey P, Knight CF. *UNIPAC Two: Alleviating Psychological and Spiritual Pain in the Terminally Ill*. American Academy of Hospice and Palliative Medicine. Dubuque, Iowa: Kendall/Hunt Publishing Company; 1997.
32. Vanderzee J. *Ministry to Persons with Chronic Illnesses* Minneapolis: Augsburg Fortress, 1993.
33. Weston J. The spiritual dimension in psychosocial assessment: a case study. *J Religion Health*. 1991; 30(3):207-213.
34. Zoloth-Dorfman L. Face to face, not eye to eye: further conversations on Jewish medical ethics. *J Clin Ethics*. 1995;Fall:222-231.

MODULE EIGHTEEN

Ethical Concepts in Hospice and Palliative Medicine

Ethical Principles

The principles outlined in the Hippocratic oath helped define medical ethics for 2500 years. With the onset of the 1900s, gradual but significant changes in medical and judicial institutions occurred. As society attempted to deal with increasingly complex medical issues, ethical decisions were no longer the implicit domain of medical professionals or the clergy. Then, during the 1980s, four basic ethical principles emerged: beneficence, nonmaleficence, autonomy, and justice.

- **Beneficence.** The principle of beneficence obliges physicians to act always in the best interests of the patient, or more explicitly, to "do good" for patients. In palliative medicine, beneficence requires the use of medical skills and knowledge to provide effective pain and symptom management, the provision of psychosocial and spiritual support, and the maintenance of dignity.
- **Nonmaleficence.** The principle of nonmaleficence denotes a responsibility to avoid doing harm to patients (*primum non nocere*), or simply, to "avoid evil." In palliative medicine , transgressions of nonmaleficence include destroying hope, failing to provide adequate opiate analgesia due to fear of precipitating death, and providing treatments when their burdens exceed benefits.

- **Autonomy.** The principle of autonomy refers to a patient's right to make decisions regarding treatment(s) according to his/her own belief system, cultural and personal values, and life plans. Or, more simply stated, one person does not have the right to make medical decisions for other people without their permission. The right to autonomy applies even when the patient's decisions differ from physicians' recommendations; moreover, disagreement about proposed medical care is not grounds for a paternalistic determination of impaired decision-making capacity. However, autonomy does not extend to the patient a right to insist that any and all treatments be provided, regardless of their likely benefits or costs. Furthermore, autonomy is limited in that its application may not impinge on the rights and freedoms of others.
- **Justice.** The principle of justice implies that physicians have an obligation to treat similar patient situations in a similar fashion. The good of society must be considered in light of finite resources, which should be equitably allocated to benefit all patients.

It is when these four principles come into conflict that much of the difficulty in ethical decision making occurs.

Decision-Making Capacity

Decision-making capacity refers to a person's ability to understand information and the implications of treatment choices, as well as to make and communicate a choice. Decision-making capacity may be temporarily compromised, fluctuate from hour to hour, or be permanently impaired. The patient's capacity to make decisions can be affected by drugs, psychological disturbances (such as depression), comorbid medical conditions, and advancing disease. Often the concept of competence is used interchangeably with decision-making capacity. However, competence refers to a person's legal status as determined by a legal authority such as a judge, and therefore is not synonymous with decision-making capacity.

A patient's decision-making capacity often is determined by the following: (1) frequent (daily) patient observations by physicians, family members, surrogates, and other health care professionals; (2) asking the patient to paraphrase topics under discussion; (3) psychiatric consultations; and (4) mental status tests such as the Folstein Mini-Mental Status Exam. However, reliance on objective tests must be tempered, because cognitively impaired patients may still be able to make decisions regarding medical care and end-of-life treatments. In fact, mental status tests typically are insensitive instruments for screening for impaired decision-making capacity, and should not be used as the sole determinant of decision-making capacity. If a patient's decision-making capacity is unclear, physicians should not make paternalistic, unilateral judgments based solely on mental status tests or personal observations. Instead, a psychiatrist or other physician skilled in determining capacity should be consulted. In addition, ethics committees may be utilized when available. Nevertheless, physicians must remember that a patient is presumed to have decision-making capacity until proven otherwise.

When a patient lacks decision-making capacity, previously expressed wishes or requests should be honored (including instructions documented in advance directives) or a designated surrogate should make decisions. However, surrogate decision makers should utilize the principles of substituted judgment and the best-interest standard when considering treatment options for the patient. Substituted judgment directs the surrogate to make decisions based on the patient's earlier statements and actions regarding choices the patient would make if currently able to formulate and express autonomous preferences. The best-interest standard requires the surrogate to make choices that maximize benefit to the patient.

Informed Consent

Informed consent is related to decision-making capacity. The purpose of informed consent is to allow a reasonable person to make autonomous treatment choices. Two conditions are involved: (1) the patient or surrogate must be competent or have decision-making capacity, which implies the ability to understand the consequences of the consent and to make decisions free from coercion or undue influence; and (2) the healthcare professional must provide necessary information in an understandable manner so valid decisions can be rendered.

Advance Directives

In 1990, the Patient Self-Determination Act was passed by Congress. It directs healthcare facilities receiving Medicaid or Medicare funds to inform patients of their right to complete an advance directive and to refuse medical treatment. Advance directives are completed when the patient has decision-making capacity, and become effective when the patient loses the ability to make decisions. Two common types of advance directives are instructive and proxy, illustrated by the Living Will and Durable Power of Attorney for Health Care, respectively.

A Durable Power of Attorney for Health Care authorizes a designated person to act as an agent or proxy to make healthcare decisions on behalf of a patient. In the absence of a Power of Attorney or healthcare surrogate, most states legislate the sequence of individuals who may act on behalf of the patient—usually the spouse, then adult children, followed by parents or siblings. Living wills are documents that may express a person's desire to die a natural death and avoid being kept alive by artificial means. Living wills usually become effective when the patient is determined to be near death. The Uniform Rights of the Terminally Ill Act (Uniform Law Commissioners, 1989) mandate the following:

1. physicians provided with a copy of a patient's living will must make it a part of the medical record;
2. verbal revocation of the will by the patient is possible at any time without regard to the patient's physical or mental condition; and
3. physicians unwilling to comply with a patient's wishes must inform the patient promptly and make all reasonable effort to transfer the patient to another health care provider.

Withholding and Withdrawing Life-Sustaining Treatment

Contrary to common belief, there is no ethical distinction between withholding and withdrawing life-sustaining treatment. Moreover, such actions are not contrary to beneficence and nonmaleficence. Withdrawing treatments at the request of competent patients is considered ethically appropriate; however, withdrawing life-sustaining therapies from incompetent patients is problematic. The Karen Ann Quinlan and Nancy Cruzan court cases affirmed that unwanted life-

sustaining treatments such as tube feedings can be withdrawn from patients in a persistent vegetative state when requested by a surrogate decision maker. When the benefits of a treatment are ambiguous, providing the treatment and then withdrawing it if it proves ineffectual is preferable to not offering the therapy due to concerns about subsequent withdrawal. Decisions to withhold or withdraw treatments should be based upon four conditions:

1. the patient's wishes,
2. medical indications,
3. the benefits and burdens of treatment, and
4. quality of life that may result from treatment.

Withholding artificial nutrition and hydration does not refer to spoon feeding or syringing fluid into a patient's mouth, but rather to treatments such as intravenous fluids and feedings, subcutaneous hydration, and tube feedings. Some states prohibit discontinuation of artificial nutrition and hydration; however, many states permit the patient's healthcare proxy (surrogate) to make decisions about withholding or withdrawing food or fluid from the patient. If artificial nutrition or hydration is provided for a patient close to death, it should meet a clearly defined therapeutic goal. Withholding or withdrawing food and fluid may result in hypernatremia, hyperosmolarity, and azotemia, which may produce a sedative effect during the dying process.

Futility

Futility is difficult to define; however, a treatment may be considered futile when, in almost all similar circumstances, it does not succeed in achieving a desired outcome. Patients or family members most often request futile interventions when they have unrealistic goals, experience feelings of guilt, have difficulty formulating a treatment plan, mistrust physicians, differ ethnically and socio-economically from healthcare professionals, deny the patient's terminal status, or have difficulty communicating due to language barriers. Physicians are not obligated to provide futile treatments or to provide treatments that violate personal or professional standards of medical practice. However, physicians should appreciate that some treatments offering little-to-no physiological benefits may provide psychological benefits and warrant a therapeutic trial.

Virtue-Based Ethics

Virtue ethics is a systematic formulation of praiseworthy character traits. Virtues which define the character of a good physician include (1) honoring the trust of the physician-patient relationship; (2) protecting the patient from exploitation and refraining from using the patient as a means of advancing power, prestige, profit, or pleasure; (3) exhibiting concern, empathy, and consideration for the patient's plight; (4) demonstrating intellectual honesty, for example, knowing when to say "I don't know"; and (5) displaying prudence.

Do Not Resuscitate

Cardiopulmonary resuscitation (CPR) was initially developed for patients with acute illness such as trauma, near-drowning, or myocardial infarction. Now CPR is frequently used to resuscitate anyone who experiences cardiopulmonary arrest. Because CPR is almost never effective or beneficial when applied to terminally ill patients, discussing a do-not-resuscitate (DNR) order with patients, surrogates and family members is vital. When discussing a DNR, physicians should provide information about the resuscitation procedure itself, the probability of its success or failure, other treatments which are not necessarily

withheld when a DNR order is in effect (e.g., antibiotics, artificial nutrition and hydration, pain and symptom management), and the ease with which a DNR order can be rescinded, that is, verbally at any time. Occasionally, patients or surrogates request CPR despite the presence of a terminal illness. In such cases, physicians should explore the reasons for requesting CPR (the patient may want to survive until a certain family member arrives), and discuss the many beneficial treatments that can be provided with or without a DNR order.

Euthanasia and Physician-Assisted Suicide

Euthanasia and physician-assisted suicide (PAS) have become polarizing and contentious issues that often dominate mainstream medical discussions. Proponents of euthanasia and PAS base their arguments on a high valuation of patient autonomy and mercy and the acknowledgment that suffering cannot be sufficiently relieved in some terminally ill patients. Opponents contend that PAS involves harm to patients, a circumstance that physicians have a professional obligation to avoid. Opponents also assert that a "slippery slope" could develop in which PAS would be allowed for non-terminal disabled individuals and "expensive" patients to lessen the financial burden for families and/or managed care organizations.

A patient's request for euthanasia or PAS should immediately stimulate discussion of the patient's underlying reasons for making the request, for example, unrelieved pain, feeling like a burden to family members, or feelings of hopelessness. Often, underlying issues can be resolved, thus eliminating the desire for suicide. In states that legalize PAS for patients, comprehensive expert palliative care should be provided before considering PAS as a last resort.

Objectives

Attitudes/Behaviors

1. Demonstrate empathy and understanding for patients who choose hospice/palliative care instead of curative care.

2. Recognize that patients and/or surrogates have a right to information about the benefits and risks/burdens of various therapeutic interventions.

3. Recognize the need for collaborative efforts when determining a patient's decision-making capacity.

4. Discuss the ethical concept that decisions to withhold or withdraw fluid and nutrition are analogous to decisions to withhold or withdraw cardiopulmonary resuscitation or dialysis.

5. Recognize the importance of exploring the reasons for a patient's wish for euthanasia or physician-assisted suicide.

6. Discuss the implications of abandonment when a physician disagrees with a patient's decision.

Knowledge

1. Define the ethical principles of beneficence, nonmaleficence, autonomy, and justice.

2. Discuss the difference between competence and decision-making capacity.

3. Define futility and its relationship to terminally ill patients.

4. Describe instructive and proxy advance directives.

5. Describe the Patient Self-Determination Act.

6. Explain how decision-making capacity is determined in a terminally ill patient.

7. Present the arguments offered by proponents and opponents of physician-assisted suicide and euthanasia.

8. Discuss virtue-based ethics.

Skills

1. Present information to patients and/or surrogates in an understandable manner so they can make educated decisions about treatments.

2. Assess patients for decision-making capacity.

3. Utilize the patient's values, goals, and priorities in medical decision making.

4. Discuss and document the rationale for decisions and orders regarding life-sustaining treatments.

5. Utilize advance directives appropriately in specific clinical scenarios.

6. Demonstrate appropriate utilization of orders not to resuscitate.

7. Demonstrate the appointment of proxy decision makers in the absence of a previously designated surrogate.

8. Demonstrate problem-solving abilities when disagreeing with a patient's decision or request.

References

1. American Thoracic Society. Withholding and withdrawing life-sustaining therapy. *Ann Intern Med*. 1991;115:478-484.
2. Byock I. Ethics from a hospice perspective. *Am J Hospice Palliat Care*. 1994;11(4):9-11.
3. Ciocon JO, Silverstone FA, Graver LM, Foley CJ. Tube feedings in elderly patients. Indications, benefits, and complications. *Arch Intern Med*. 1988;148:429-433.
4. *Deciding To Forego Life-Sustaining Treatment*. Washington, DC: President's Commission for the Study of Ethical Problems in Medicine and Biomedical and Behavioral Research; March, 1983.
5. Ethics Committee of the Society of Critical Care Medicine. Consensus statement of the Society of Critical Care Medicine's ethics committee regarding futile and other possibly inadvisable treatment. *Crit Care Med*. 1997;25(5):887-891.
6. Fins JJ. Futility in clinical practice: report on a congress of clinical societies. *J Am Geriatr Soc*. 1994;42:861-865.
7. Garrett TM, Baillie HW, Garrett RM. *Health Care Ethics: Principles and Problems*. Englewood Cliffs, NJ: Prentice Hall, 1993.
8. Hardwig J. Is there a duty to die? *Hastings Cen Report*. 1997;27(2):34-42.
9. Jonsen AR, Siegler M, Winslade WJ. *Clinical Ethics*. New York: Macmillan Publishing, 1982.
10. Kinzbrunner BM. Ethical dilemmas in hospice and palliative care. *Support Care Cancer*. 1995; 3:28-36.
11. Moulin DE, Latimer EJ, MacDonald N, et al. Statement on euthanasia and physician-assisted suicide. *J Palliat Care*. 1994;10(2):80-81.
12. Orentlicher D. Advance medical directives. *JAMA*. 1990;263:2365-2367.
13. Peabody FW. The care of the patient. *JAMA*. 1927;88:877-882.
14. Pellegrino ED. The metamorphosis of medical ethics. *JAMA*. 1993;269:1158-1162.
15. Printz LA. Terminal dehydration, a compassionate treatment. *Arch Intern Med*. 1992;152:697-700.
16. Report of the Task Force on Physician-Assisted Suicide of the Society for Health and Human Values. Physician-assisted suicide: toward a comprehensive understanding. *Acad Med*. 1995; 5:583-590.
17. Scanlon C, Fleming C. Ethical issues in caring for the patient with advanced cancer. *Nurs Clin North Am*. 1989;24:977-986.
18. Scott JF, Lynch J. Bedside assessment of competency in palliative care. *J Palliat Care*. 1994;10(3):101-105.
19. Stanley, JM, ed. The Appleton international conference: developing guidelines for decisions to forgo life-prolonging medical treatment. *J Med Ethics*. 1992;18:3-22. (suppl)
20. Storey P, Knight CF. *UNIPAC Six: Ethical and Legal Decision Making When Caring for the Terminally Ill*. American Academy of Hospice and Palliative Medicine. Dubuque, Iowa: Kendall/Hunt Publishing Company; 1996.
21. The Hastings Center. *Guidelines on the Termination of Life-Sustaining Treatment and the Care of the Dying*. Bloomington, Indiana: Indiana University Press; 1987.
22. Tomlinson T, Brody H. Futility and the ethics of resuscitation. *JAMA*. 1990;264:1276-1280.
23. Wanzer SH, Federman DD, Adelstein SJ, et al. The physician's responsibility toward hopelessly ill patients: a second look. *N Engl J Med*. 1989;329:844-849.
24. Weir RF. The morality of physician-assisted suicide. *Law, Medicine, and Health Care*. 1992; 20:116-126.
25. Wilkinson J. The ethics of communication in palliative care. *Palliat Care* .1991;5:130-137.
26. Wilkinson J. Ethical issues in palliative care. In: Doyle D, Hanks GWC, MacDonald N, eds. *Oxford Textbook of Palliative Medicine*. Oxford: Oxford University Press; 1993:495-504.

MODULE NINETEEN

The Process of Dying and Managing the Death Event

The physician's role during and immediately after the death of a patient varies from serving as a close mentor and guide, to providing orders, prescriptions, and follow-up with staff and bereaved family members. Understanding the physiology of the dying process is likely to increase physician comfort and competence when serving as a mentor and when managing the death event.

Rarely is it necessary or appropriate to monitor electrolytes, chemistry profiles, or blood gases in terminally ill patients who choose hospice care. However, understanding the respiratory changes associated with acidosis, the metabolic consequences of renal shut-down, and the neurologic manifestations of decorticate and decerebrate brain function can improve physician competence when predicting the time of death and when explaining visible physical changes in a patient's condition to family members and caregivers.

Physiological Changes Near the End of Life

The exact nature and sequence of physiological changes varies depending on the underlying disease and other comorbid conditions. Regardless of diagnosis, common physiological changes include alterations in respiration, mental status, circulation, and skin color.

Shortness of breath and progressive respiratory impairment can be frightening and uncomfortable for patients and family members. When physicians anticipate and understand changes in respiration, they are more likely to provide effective treatments, reassurance, and much-needed education.

Patients with pleural effusions or central obstructing lung cancers may be most comfortable sitting upright with legs dependent or leaning over a table or chair. Such postures permit maximum use of accessory neck and chest muscles. As patients become weaker, positioning becomes less feasible and dyspnea is best relieved with morphine and benzodiazepines.

As death approaches, declining levels of consciousness and respiratory changes commonly occur. Patients are likely to experience irregular patterns of breathing such as Cheyne-Stokes respiration, agonal respiration, and periods of apnea, which often appear several days prior to death and increase in frequency and length until the patient dies. Cheyne-Stokes respiration is characterized by increasingly rapid respirations alternating with intervals of apnea. Agonal respirations occur in deeply comatose patients and are characterized by regular, shallow, labored, open-mouth breathing requiring much respiratory effort.

As patients become weaker and increasingly obtunded, often they are no longer able to clear secretions effectively. Secretions may pool in the posterior pharynx, creating a gurgling sound often referred to as the "death rattle." Suctioning irritates the patient's airways; more effective and humane treatments include repositioning, coupled with use of anticholinergics such as scopolamine or hyoscamine to decrease secretions. Throughout the dying process, family members and caregivers can provide mouth care, which benefits the patient and involves the family in active expressions of caring and nurturing.

Most patients experience circulatory changes prior to death. As cardiac output drops, baroreceptors cause decreased blood flow to the extremities to preserve vital organ functions. The patient's nailbeds, knees, and even the tip of the nose may become cyanotic or mottled. Discoloration is accompanied by progressive coolness of the extremities, which usually predicts death within a few days. Loss of a palpable radial pulse may indicate death within hours. In addition, as death approaches, urinary output drops precipitously due to decreased intake of food and fluids and diminished blood flow to the kidneys.

As patients receive less oral intake, third space fluids will be reabsorbed. Patients with peripheral edema, ascites, and other third space fluids may reabsorb the fluids back into circulation, which can sustain life after parenteral fluids have been withdrawn. Decreased peripheral edema may contribute to the patient's comfort due to decreasing tissue distention. Resorption of ascites or pleural effusions may reduce respiratory difficulty resulting from pulmonary restriction.

Urinary incontinence usually occurs as patients become progressively weaker and their mental status declines. Urinary retention also may occur, usually requiring a Foley catheter to improve comfort and protect skin from maceration and breakdown.

The gradual dehydration that often occurs prior to death does not always result in diminished mental status or coma. In at least two circumstances, steady decreases in oral intake

and fluid volume result in temporary increases in the patient's alertness. Patients with primary and metastatic brain tumors may exhibit transient improvements in mental status when global dehydration reduces edema associated with central lesions. When patients with end-stage liver disease decrease their consumption of fluids and protein-containing foods, they may experience decreased ascites and hepatic congestion, as well as reduced ammonia levels and subsequent improvement in associated hepatic encephalopathy. Physicians should explain these temporary and confusing "improvements" in mental status to families and caregivers.

Symptom Relief Near the End of Life

Whenever possible, physicians, patients, nurses, and family members should openly discuss the management of terminal symptoms. The goals of treatment must be clearly defined and reviewed frequently. Treatments such as artificial hydration and nutrition and transfusions, which may have provided significant benefit in the past, are likely to become burdensome as the disease progresses.

When patients lose the ability to swallow, families frequently struggle with issues such as withholding or withdrawing parenteral hydration and nutrition. Physicans should explain the dying process and the potential metabolic burdens associated with artificial hydration and nutrition in terminally ill patients. Education also can help patients and family members make educated choices and may relieve their fears about "starving" a loved one.

When the stress of waiting for death to occur is perceived as overwhelming, some patients and family members may request hastened death. Clear and compassionate explanations of the goals of palliative care, which do not include prolonging life or hastening death, can be reassuring. In addition to providing education, physicians must attend to all of the details of care to ensure maximal patient comfort.

It is imperative to provide family members and caregivers with psychological support and education and to encourage periodic breaks from the demands of caregiving. Unalterable decisions made when families and caregivers are deeply fatigued may not be in the patient's best interests. Few decisions at the end of life can be considered wrong if made in the best interests of the patient. The astute medical professional recognizes the ethical and moral struggles confronted by patients and family members. Expert clinical interventions, ongoing support, flexibility, and ethical decision making are paramount.

As death approaches and patients enter the active phase of dying, continued symptom relief is crucial. (See other modules for specific treatments—module 6 for pain, module 9 for dyspnea, and module 10 for nausea and vomiting.) Because most patients lose the ability to swallow, physicians must be skilled in administering medications via alternative routes and adjusting medication dosages as needed. Previously controlled symptoms may crescendo just before death; thus, physicians should anticipate the need for urgent palliation with proactive interventions.

Careful planning and expert symptom control usually obviate the need for intravenous treatments, which are rarely indicated or advantageous for patients who are dying. Inserting intravenous needles usually is painful, particularly in dehydrated patients, and additional fluids may create new symptoms and prolong the dying process. The gadgetry of intravenous infusion systems is likely to further stress patients and families, who are already under significant duress. Administering concentrated solutions via buccal or sublingual routes is preferred. When subcutaneous infusions are necessary, use a 25-gauge butterfly needle hooked to a syringe driver or small computerized pump. Many analgesics and sedatives also can be given rectally.

When patients become comatose, the primary focus of care continues to be comfort. Pain medications should continue around the clock, with adjustments as needed to relieve distress indicated by non-verbal signs. Pre-treatment to relieve pain associated with turning, bathing, and changing clothing or linens can be advantageous. Medications for treating chronic diseases such as diabetes or hypertension can be discontinued at this time.

Some symptoms may be more distressing for family members and caregivers than for patients. Restlessness from organ failure-related encephalopathy may be more difficult to observe than to experience. Patients frequently experience restlessness just prior to death. However, when restlessness occurs, careful assessments should rule out underlying causes such as obstipation, full bladder, or pain. When severe restlessness occurs, safety concerns may require gentle sedation to achieve light sleep. Ideally, sedation should be discussed with family members and with patients before decision-making capacity is compromised.

Some patients experience agitated delirium, which is characterized by more intense symptoms than simple restlessness. Frequently, delirium jeopardizes the ability of family members to care for patients at home. Medications such as haloperidol or chlorpromazine commonly are prescribed to relieve delirium. However haloperidol and morphine can also *cause* delirium, making thorough reassessments critical. Some patients experience extreme death-related anxiety, due perhaps to insufficient opportunity or means to resolve painful emotional, social, or spiritual issues. The hospice interdisciplinary team approach to care provides an ideal method for involving patients, family members, and caregivers in identifying and relieving sources of emotional and spiritual suffering earlier in the course of the illness. When all other treatments fail, sedation with infusions of midazolam or barbiturates may be the only means of providing comfort and relief from symptoms.

Restlessness and delirium should not be confused with myoclonus, which is characterized by random twitching or jerking of extremities that is sometimes confused with seizure activity. Myoclonus is most often associated with high doses of opioids and hepatic or renal failure. Myoclonus significantly exacerbates pain in patients with widespread bone metastases. Liberal dosing with benzodiazepines or barbiturates usually is necessary to quiet involuntary movements, and a continuous infusion may be required. Relieving restlessness, agitation, and severe myoclonus has profound effects on the deathbed experience for patients and family members. When these very distressing symptoms are effectively managed, survivors are more likely to remember their loved one's death as peaceful and may be able to negotiate the bereavement process with fewer difficulties.

Non-drug interventions such as massage, music, fans, soothing touch, and talk are important adjunct therapies that may help alleviate anxiety and restlessness. During the dying process, imagery and distraction may not be as effective due to changes in mental status that impede the patient's ability to participate.

Oral swabbing with water or soda water improves hygiene and soothes dry mucous membranes. Artificial tears can provide soothing relief when a patient's eyes do not completely close and the blink reflex stops. Gentle massage may ease stiffness and discomfort.

Involving family members, friends, and caregivers in the patient's care helps ensure the provision of appropriate interventions and improves the level of care. Typically, family members and friends welcome opportunities to care for patients as death occurs. Involving them in active care often promotes a greater sense of contributing to the patient's comfort, which may lead to an easier bereavement.

Physician Involvement Near the End of Life

Physicians play a crucial role as educators and guides through the last days and hours of a patient's life. Families and patients look to physicians for guidance regarding length of life, not only in terms of finalizing business and legal matters but also in terms of personal closure. Thus, physicians frequently are asked to predict the patient's time of death. Unfortunately, prognostication is difficult. Little data exists regarding the prognosis of patients receiving palliative therapies, and the results of population-based studies cannot be directly applied to individual cases.

Earlier in the course of a patient's illness, attempts to prognosticate a specific number of weeks or months of life are fraught with difficulty; and physicians often are proved wrong, particularly when prognosticating the length of life for patients with non-cancer diseases. As the illness progresses, physicians often can provide benchmarks that allow patients and families to make necessary plans for the future and focus on issues of particular importance. When death approaches, a patient's length of life may be more predictable in terms of hours to days or days to weeks, based on diagnosis, rate of decline, functional and nutritional status, and physiological changes.

Throughout the dying process, patients and families may struggle with psychological and spiritual issues that are at least as distressing as the physical aspects of illness and decline. Patients often become frustrated or depressed about their increasing dependence. They may withdraw socially or express anger and bitterness at loved ones, which can be terribly distressing for family members and friends who have gathered to provide physical care and emotional support. Occasionally, patients are so distressed, family members become fearful.

As issues arise, physicians should involve other healthcare professionals, such as a social worker, a counselor, or a chaplain as soon as possible to address the situation and to facilitate resolution of tensions and/or unspoken or unfinished personal issues. Other team members may be more familiar with the patient's and family's specific issues and thus be better equipped to address them.

The interdisciplinary team approach to care facilitates and supports the creation of a healing environment, which is crucial to the patient's continued personal growth, spiritual expression, and emotional healing during the dying process. Thus, the notion of a "good death" can be understood in terms of the subjective experiences of both the patient and family. Dying well is often associated with a sense of renewed purpose, hope, fulfillment, and completion at the end of life. The realization that continued emotional and spiritual growth is possible in the midst of physical decline can be profoundly meaningful for patients and family members.

As patients become progressively weaker, physicians and nurses can serve as role models for family members and caregivers by attending to the details of care, ensuring the patient's comfort, communicating compassionately and honestly, and providing education, reassurance, and ongoing emotional support for family members as they care for the dying patient.

Physicians must maintain vigilance regarding pain and symptom relief. Effectively controlling symptoms improves the patient's physical comfort and reduces the patient's and family's anxiety about potential physical suffering during the death event. As death approaches, physicians should give family members permission to stay by the patient's bedside as long as they wish, to express final words of love, to hold the patient's hand, and to sing and pray together.

Frequently, patients die when neither the physician nor family members are present. Even for families in vigil, death often occurs when family members have left the room, even briefly. In such cases, family members may react intensely, verbalizing a profound sense of failure for not being present at the moment of death. Physicians can do much to relieve potential anguish by mentioning this phenomenon, by explaining that some patients seem to prefer to die alone, and by providing ongoing reassurance after death occurs. After the patient dies, family members should be given permission to remain with the body as long as desired and to clean the body if they wish to do so.

After the patient's death, physicians have ongoing responsibilities. Timely and accurate completion of the death certificate is crucial; the document is necessary for cremation or burial, and provides survivors with the proof of death to resolve legal and business affairs. Physicians should be knowledgeable about state requirements regarding death certification.

Physician involvement during bereavement varies. When physicians have long-term relationships with a patient and family, they may be included in personal and community expressions of loss. Providing continued opportunities for families to ask questions, even for months after the death, can be very helpful for survivors. Hospice programs are required to provide ongoing bereavement services for family members for at least a year after the patient's death.

Physicians are privileged to care for patients throughout the dying process and to be present at the time of death. However, the emotional and spiritual impact of caring for terminally ill patients should not be discounted, particularly when the patient's death ends a long-term patient/physician relationship. Acknowledging feelings of grief, using stress management techniques, and taking as many short breaks as possible can help physicians cope with the inevitable stresses that accompany compassionate care of people who are dying.

Objectives

Attitudes/Behaviors

1. Display comfort at the bedside of an actively dying patient.

2. Defend the active nature of palliative care before, during, and after a patient's death.

3. Respect the differing needs of patients and families throughout the dying process.

4. Display concern for the continued comfort of patients who can no longer communicate their needs.

5. Discuss the importance of controlling patients' symptoms near the end of life.

6. Describe the importance of preventive medical care near the end of life.

7. Display professional vigilance for meeting the ongoing needs of patients when life-prolonging or curative therapies are no longer indicated or desired.

8. Display respect for patients during the dying process.

Knowledge

1. Discuss and interpret the pathophysiologic relationships between organ failure of the heart, lungs, brain, and kidneys, and the process of dying.

2. Describe key components of home care for terminally ill patients, including symptom management and the provision of emotional and spiritual support for patients and family members.

3. Describe physiological signs of approaching death, including changes in breathing patterns, decreased levels of consciousness, mottling of the skin, and coolness of the extremities, and discuss their likely implications for prognosis in terms of hours and days.

4. Discuss options for care settings during the dying process and describe indications for transferring patients from one setting to another.

5. Describe methods for helping families cope with the physical and psychological changes that accompany the death event.

6. Discuss indications and contraindications for the following treatments for terminally ill patients, including impact on prognosis: transfusions, routes of medication administration, nutritional support, hydration, and withholding and withdrawing treatments.

7. Discuss effective oral and ocular care during the dying process.

8. Explain the appropriateness of discontinuing medications not essential for physical comfort, such as antihypertensives, cardiac drugs, or antidiabetic agents.

9. Describe signs of approaching death and post-mortem changes.

10. Describe the following physiologic crises, which commonly occur near death, the predisposing characteristics, and treatments for each: delirium, severe dyspnea, and seizures.

11. Explain appropriate physician roles following a patient's death, whether at home or an inpatient setting.

12. Explain family support needs during and after a patient's death.

13. Differentiate religion and spirituality.

14. Explain common spiritual issues that accompany terminal illness, and describe interventions for alleviating spiritual pain.

Skills

1. Demonstrate effective application of hospice care principles when caring for terminally ill patients, including use of the interdisciplinary team approach to care.

2. Manage the following signs and symptoms of impending death: the "death rattle," massive hemorrhage, changing levels of consciousness, mottling and cooling of the extremities, altered respiratory patterns, myoclonus, terminal agitation, and delirium.

3. Provide adequate pain and symptom management in a patient who cannot swallow.

4. Provide education and emotional support for family members during the dying process.

5. Validate appropriate family decisions and the family's efforts on behalf of the patient.

6. Accurately complete a death certificate using the appropriate cause of death.

7. Use education and supportive interventions to prepare families and friends psychologically for the patient's death.

References

1. Bottomley DM, Hanks GW. Subcutaneous midazolam infusion in palliative care. *J Pain Symptom Manage.* 1990;5:259-261.
2. Breitbart W, Bruera E, Chochinov H, Lynch M. Neuropsychiatric syndromes and psychological symptoms in patients with advanced cancer. *J Pain Symptom Manage.* 1995;10(2):131-141.
3. Brody, H, Campbell, ML, Faber-Landendoen K, Ogle, KS. Withdrawing intensive life-sustaining treatment—recommendations for compassionate clinical management. *N Engl J Med.* 1997;336:652-657.
4. Byock I. *Dying Well.* New York: Riverhead Books; 1977.
5. Cherny NI, Portenoy RK. Sedation in the management of refractory symptoms: guidelines for evaluation and treatment. *J Palliat Care.* 1994;10(2):31-39.
6. Coyle N, Adelhardt J, Foley K, Portenoy R. Character of terminal illness in the advanced cancer patient: pain and other symptoms during the last four weeks of life. *J Pain Symptom Manage.* 1990;5:83-93.
7. Greene W, Davis W. Titrated IV barbiturates in the control of symptoms in patients with terminal cancer. *South Med J.* 1991;84:332-227.

8. Hentleff, P. Dyspnea management: to take into the air my quiet breath. *Palliat Care*. 1898;5:52-54.
9. Kaye P. *Notes on Symptom Control in Hospice and Palliative Care*. Essex, Connecticut: Hospice Education Institution; 1989.
10. McCann RM, Hall W, Groth-Junker A. Comfort care for terminally ill patients, the appropriate use of nutrition and hydration. *JAMA*. 1994;272:1263-1266.
11. McCue, J. The naturalness of dying. *JAMA*. 1995;273:1039-1043.
12. Morita T, et al. Sedation for symptom control in Japan: the importance of intermittent use and communication with family members. *J Pain Symptom Manage*. 1996;12:32-38.
13. Storey P, Hill H, St. Louis RH, Tarver EE. Subcutaneous infusions for control of cancer symptoms. *J Pain Symptom Manage*. 1990;5:33-41.
14. Strause L, Herbst L, Ryndes T. A severity index designed as an indicator of acuity in palliative care. *J Palliat Care*. 1993;9(4):11-15.
15. Truog RD, Berde CB, Mitchell C, Grier HE. Barbiturates in the care of the terminally ill. *New Engl J Med*. 1992;327:1678-1682.
16. Twycross RG, Lichter I. The terminal phase. In: Doyle D, Hanks, GWC, MacDonald N, eds. *Oxford Textbook of Palliative Medicine*. New York: Oxford University Press: 1993; 651-661.
17. Ventafridda, et al. Symptom prevalence and control during cancer patients' last days of life. *J Palliat Care*. 1990;6:7-11.

Financing Hospice and Palliative Medicine

Economics of End-of-Life Care

Medical care at the end of life is responsible for approximately 10 percent to 12 percent of the total healthcare budget. About 27 percent of the Medicare budget (approximately $45 billion in 1994) is spent on end-of-life care, with Medicare expenditures specifically for hospice care totaling only about 2.6 percent of that amount ($1.2 billion in 1994).

Initial studies evaluating the cost effectiveness of hospice care suggested that hospice programs provided useful services at lower costs than conventional care. Subsequently, in 1982, Congress authorized the Medicare Hospice Benefit (MHB), one of the country's earliest managed care reimbursement systems. Studies later reported that the benefit's impact on overall healthcare costs was unclear or, at best, minimal.

More recently, a study commissioned by the National Hospice Organization demonstrated that for every dollar Medicare spent on hospice, the Medicare program saved $1.52. The study also showed that patients electing the MHB incurred $2,737 less in healthcare costs during the last year of life than those not receiving hospice care prior to death. A more recent study, published in 1996, analyzed existing data on the costs of hospice and other forms of end-of-life care. The results of the study suggested that hospice may save 10 percent to 17 percent of the healthcare costs incurred during the last six months of life,

with the greatest savings occurring during the last month of life.

Analysis of available data suggests that the MHB provides cost-effective, end-of-life care to terminally ill patients and their families. However, the benefit has had minimal effect on overall national healthcare expenditures, due primarily to the fact that most eligible patients do not receive hospice services. Demographic data show that only about 50 percent of terminally ill cancer patients and only about 17 percent of all dying patients receive hospice services. Of patients who do receive hospice care, reported lengths of stay indicate that referrals may occur so late in the illness trajectory, patients and families may not benefit fully from hospice services. Hospice providers and the medical community must work together to overcome barriers to hospice care, thus allowing patients and families not only to take full advantage of the MHB but also to receive the high quality and potentially cost-effective palliative care services to which they are entitled.

Palliative Care Services for Non-Terminal Patients

While the concepts and goals of hospice care and palliative care are similar, reimbursement is very different. When the government developed the MHB, it provided a unique managed care reimbursement system which allowed hospice programs to provide palliative care for eligible patients during the last six months of life. However, palliative care for non-terminal patients continues to be reimbursed by traditional resources. Consequently, traditional healthcare providers, such as home health agencies and hospitals, must provide palliative care for patients who are not eligible for the MHB. Because patients receiving services from traditional providers must meet demanding admission criteria, health care professionals may be forced to limit palliative care services provided to non-hospice patients.

To implement their mission and provide palliative care for patients not meeting the MHB eligibility requirements, some hospices have established creative "bridge programs" to fill the gap between home health care and hospice care. The effects of changes in reimbursement for home health services on a hospice program's ability to provide palliative services for patients prior to their eligibility for hospice remain unclear.

Recognizing the potential importance of palliative care in mainstream medicine, the Health Care Financing Administration (HCFA) is currently testing a Diagnosis Related Group (DRG) modifier for palliative care. The effects and outcomes of the modifier are not yet fully understood.

The Medicare Hospice Benefit

Since the MHB was authorized in 1982, it has allowed hospice programs to provide comprehensive palliative care for thousands of terminally ill patients and their families. The benefit also defined patient eligibility, established conditions of participation, including where and how care can be delivered, and created a reimbursement structure that encouraged hospice programs to accept fiscal as well as healthcare management responsibility. The Medicare Hospice benefit also served as a

model for most states' Medicaid Hospice Benefit and for the hospice benefits offered by increasing numbers of private insurance carriers and managed care plans. Therefore, a thorough knowledge of the MHB is essential for understanding the financing of palliative care for most terminally ill patients.

Patient Eligibility

To qualify for the MHB, patients must meet the following criteria: (1) eligibility for Medicare Part A, which provides patients with hospital insurance coverage; (2) certification of terminal illness, that is, two physicians must certify the patient's prognosis as six months or less, if the terminal illness runs its normal course; (3) choice of the MHB by giving informed consent and signing a document to that effect; and (4) care for the terminal illness must be provided by a Medicare-certified hospice program. When patients are certified as terminally ill, one of the certifying physicians must be the patient's attending physician and the other must be the hospice medical director (or his/her designee). Certification must be provided orally within two days of admission and in writing prior to the hospice's billing Medicare for services. (See Module 15 for a description of guidelines for determining a prognosis of six months or less in non-cancer patients.)

Benefit Periods

The original MHB provided reimbursement for hospice programs for up to 210 days of care, which were divided into three benefit periods—two 90-day periods and a final 30-day period. Since then, the benefit has been modified twice and now consists of two 90-day periods followed by an unlimited number of 60-day benefit periods. The changes were instituted to safeguard a patient's eligibility for covered hospice services regardless of length of life, as long as the patient continues to be certified as terminally ill.

Reimbursement for Hospice Services

As with other managed care programs, hospice programs are reimbursed on a per diem basis. In this case, the government pays the hospice a fixed daily rate for each patient under its care. Hospice programs then use the per diem payment to provide all services necessary to palliate symptoms related to the patient's terminal condition. The scope of services hospice programs are required to provide is extensive and includes medical services (in coordination with the attending physician), nursing services, home health aide services, psychosocial and spiritual support services, bereavement counseling for up to one year after the patient dies, drugs and biologicals necessary to treat the terminal illness and its symptoms, medical supplies and durable medical equipment (DME), physical therapy, occupational therapy, speech therapy, and dietary counseling as indicated by the patient's plan of care.

Unlike other Medicare benefits, which generally are reimbursed at 80 percent (i.e., they require a 20 percent co-payment by the patient), the MHB is essentially a 100 percent benefit. In most cases, patients do not incur any out-of-pocket expenses for hospice services provided under the MHB, as long as the services are required to palliate the symptoms secondary to the terminal condition and are included in the patient's plan of care. Hospice programs may charge patients a 5 percent co-payment for each day of respite care and for prescription medications, with the latter limited to a maximum of $5 per prescription; however, most hospices do not attempt to collect these co-payments.

The MHB established per diem rates, which are based on geographic economic factors, to reimburse hospice programs for the four levels of care required by the MHB—routine home care, continuous home care, respite inpatient care, and general inpatient care. Routine home care is basic care provided in the patient's home; currently it is reimbursed at about $90 to $100 per day.

Continuous care is provided for patients wishing to remain at home instead of being transferred to an acute care setting during times of crisis. Crises usually occur secondary to acute medical symptoms. To be eligible for continuous care, patients must require primarily nursing services (a minimum of 51 percent of the care must be provided by a registered nurse) and must need continuous care for a minimum of eight hours a day. Currently, reimbursement for continuous care is about $25 per hour, or approximately $600 for 24 hours.

Inpatient respite care is most commonly used when a patient's family needs relief from the day-to-day responsibilities of caring for the patient at home. Respite care is provided when patients need an inpatient environment but do not meet the requirements for general inpatient care, as described below. Respite care is limited to five consecutive days per stay and is reimbursed at a rate only slightly higher than routine home care, currently between $93 and $103 per day.

General inpatient care is available for procedures necessary for pain control or other symptom management that cannot feasibly be provided in other settings. In 1993, the criteria for general inpatient care were revised to include a breakdown in the patient's home environment as an additional indication for general inpatient care. Hospice programs must provide access to general inpatient care when needed, as patients electing the MHB are no longer covered by Medicare Part A for acute care hospitalization. General inpatient care may be provided in a number of different settings, including hospitals, skilled nursing facilities, free-standing hospice inpatient units, or dedicated hospice inpatient units in nursing homes and hospitals. When hospice programs do not have access to dedicated inpatient units, they contract directly with hospitals or skilled nursing facilities to provide acute care on an as-needed basis. Currently, hospices are reimbursed approximately $450 for a day of general inpatient care.

Patients residing in long-term or assisted-care facilities are eligible for the MHB, just as patients living in their own homes, and are entitled to the same array of benefits and levels of care. With one exception, hospice programs providing care for patients residing in nursing facilities receive identical reimbursement as that received for providing routine care in a patient's own home. The exception is reimbursement for Medicaid patients covered by traditional Medicaid for care in a nursing facility. (See Unified Rate Reimbursement.)

The MHB was designed with safeguards to reduce the risk of over-utilization of services. Reimbursement to hospice providers is limited by what is described as a *global cap*. Hospice providers may not receive average reimbursement per patient per year in excess of the cap amount. In 1983, the cap amount was set at $6,500 per patient per year but it has since increased to about $14,000. The cap represents approximately 95 percent of the dollar amount that traditional Medicare spends on care during the last six weeks of life.

Waiver of Medicare Benefits and Coverage of Unrelated Conditions

With the exception of professional services provided by their attending physician, patients electing the MHB waive their right to coverage by traditional Medicare for services related to the treatment of their terminal condition, or for a related condition. This explains why hospices must provide access to inpatient care and other services normally covered by the Medicare program.

By inference, the waiver has been interpreted as indicating that patients requiring services for treatment of a condition unrelated to their terminal illness would be covered by regular Medicare. Therefore, such treatments would not be the financial responsibility of the hospice. The following scenario is used as an example of the shared responsibilities of care: a terminally ill hospice patient who has

elected the MHB and is receiving care from a Medicare-certified hospice program is in an automobile accident; the hospice program would continue to pay for care related to the terminal illness, but traditional Medicare Part A would cover the cost of care related to the automobile accident. Unfortunately, there is a lack of clear definition about which conditions are considered either related or unrelated to a specific terminal condition. Therefore, the hospice medical director must become intimately involved in determining which symptoms or conditions are related to a patient's terminal illness.

Revocation of the Medicare Hospice Benefit

Patients retain their right to revoke hospice care after they elect the MHB. To ensure the protection of a patient's rights, the patient may revoke the MHB at any time. Unlike most Medicare risk plans, when hospice patients revoke the MHB, they are immediately eligible for coverage by their traditional Medicare benefits, thus ensuring that they will have full Medicare coverage for any health care they require. Hospice programs may not revoke patients; however, a hospice provider may discharge a patient, for example, when the patient can no longer be certified as terminally ill due to an extended prognosis.

Physician Services

Reimbursement of physician services varies depending on the physician's role. Attending physicians who are not employees of a hospice program may bill for professional services under Medicare Part B, as usual. They receive 80 percent of the usual and customary fee from Medicare, with the other 20 percent coming either from secondary insurance or from the patient. Under current Medicare regulations, attending physicians also may bill for care plan oversight, with reimbursement dependent on documentation of their activities and time spent during the month of service billed. Other services provided by attending physicians for hospice patients, such as laboratory studies, x-rays, and medications, are not typically reimbursable under Medicare Part B. If such services are part of the hospice patient's care plan, the hospice program is responsible for the services. If such services are unrelated to the patient's terminal condition, they are reimbursable under Medicare Part B, as usual.

Consulting physicians who provide services for hospice patients for conditions related to the terminal illness must be reimbursed directly by the hospice. The MHB allows hospice programs to bill Medicare Part A on a fee-for-service basis for direct patient care services provided by a consultant; however, the consultant physician must have a contract with the hospice and the services provided must be included in the patient's plan of care. The hospice program bills Medicare Part A, which reimburses the program for consultant physician services at 100 percent of the usual and customary charge (no deductible). The hospice then pays the consultant physician.

Direct patient care services provided by Hospice Medical Directors and hospice physicians may be recouped by the hospice in the same fashion as for consultant physicians. A physician's contract with the hospice program stipulates whether the hospice remunerates the physician directly for services provided or uses generated revenues to offset the physician's salary. Routine administrative activities provided by Hospice Medical Directors and hospice physicians are covered by the per diem and are not independently reimbursable. Such activities include interdisciplinary team participation, care planning (hospice medical directors and physicians may not bill for care planning oversight for hospice patients), quality improvement, and education.

Unified Rate Reimbursement

Some patients are eligible for both Medicare and Medicaid; for example, Medicare patients living in long-term care facilities whose room and board are paid for by the Medicaid program. Hospice program reimbursement for caring for dually eligible patients is somewhat unique. Recognizing that certain services provided by the hospice and the long-term facility might be perceived as duplicative, a unified rate of reimbursement was established. The hospice provider is reimbursed both the hospice per diem rate and 95 percent of the room and board rate that Medicaid would normally pay to the long-term care facility. The hospice program is then responsible for contracting with and reimbursing the nursing facility for the patient's room and board.

Objectives

Attitudes/Behaviors

1. Describe how the Medicare Hospice Benefit has influenced the delivery of hospice and end-of-life care in the United States.

2. Discuss how the eligibility requirements for hospice care may affect patient access to care at the end of life.

3. Describe how per diem reimbursement under the Medicare Hospice Benefit may affect patient care decisions.

4. Describe how the Medicare hospice global cap helps limit improper utilization of hospice services.

5. Discuss the rationale for the current structure of the benefit periods under the Medicare Hospice Benefit.

6. Explain the importance of receiving input from the attending physician and all members of the interdisciplinary team when recertifying a patient.

7. Discuss the rationale for providing hospice services to patients living in long-term care facilities.

8. Explain the importance of Medical Director involvement in decisions related to the provision of services unrelated to the terminal condition.

9. Discuss the cost effectiveness of hospice care.

10. Discuss the limitations of the Medicare Hospice Benefit on the provision of care and the cost of care at the end of life.

Knowledge

1. Differentiate between reimbursement under traditional Medicare Part A and reimbursement under the Medicare Hospice Benefit.

2. Describe the major features of the Medicare Hospice Benefit.

3. List the four levels of hospice care under the Medicare Hospice Benefit.

4. Describe the services that a hospice must provide under per diem reimbursement by Medicare.

5. Describe the historical evolution of the Medicare Hospice Benefit.

6. Discuss the indications for general acute inpatient care and the different venues in which it may be provided.

7. Discuss the indications and reimbursement requirements for continuous care under the Medicare Hospice Benefit.

8. Discuss the concept of an unrelated condition and how it relates to the Medicare Hospice Benefit.

9. Explain when and how a patient may revoke the Medicare Hospice Benefit.

10. Explain when a hospice program may discharge a patient.

11. Discuss the different ways physicians may be reimbursed for services provided to patients under the Medicare Hospice Benefit.

12. List the services provided by the Hospice Medical Director that are covered by Medicare Hospice Benefit per diem.

13. Discuss some of the barriers to hospice services.

14. Discuss the economics of end-of-life care and its impact on the Medicare Hospice Benefit.

15. Discuss reimbursement for palliative care services for patients who are not certified as terminally ill.

Skills

1. Explain to an attending physician the process of referring patients for hospice care and the mechanism for receiving reimbursement for services provided to hospice patients.

2. Explain to a consulting physician the reimbursement process for providing services to a hospice patient.

3. Explain to a referring physician the responsibility for certifying and recertifying a patient's eligibility for the Medicare Hospice Benefit.

4. Utilize the interdisciplinary team and attending physician when evaluating patients for recertification.

5. Utilize in an appropriate manner the four levels of care for patients receiving hospice services.

6. Describe to the Medical Director of a long-term care facility the appropriate role of hospice in the care patients residing in long-term care facilities.

7. Assess whether specific treatments are related or unrelated to the terminal condition.

8. Work with community physicians and other referral sources to improve patient access to hospice programs.

References

1. A controlled trial to improve care for seriously ill hospitalized patients. The study to understand prognoses and preferences for outcomes and risks of treatments (SUPPORT). The Support Principal Investigators. *JAMA*. 1995;274:1591-1598.
2. Billings JA, Block S: Palliative care in undergraduate medical education. Status report and future directions. *JAMA*. 1997;278:733.
3. Brody H, Lynn J: The physician's responsibility under the new Medicare reimbursement for hospice care. *New Engl J Med*. 1984;310:920.
4. Cassel CK, Vladeck BC. Sounding Board. ICD-9 code for palliative or terminal care. *New Engl J Med*. 1996;335:1232-1234.
5. Christakis NA, Escarce JJ. Survival of Medicare patients after enrollment on a hospice program. *New Engl J Med*. 1996;335:172.
6. Demer C, Johnston-Anderson AV, Tobin R, et al. Cost of hospice care: late versus early entry, abstract 396. *Proceedings ASCO*. 1992;11:392.
7. Emanuel EJ. Cost savings at the end of life. What do the data show? *JAMA*. 1996;275:1907-1914.
8. Emanuel EJ, Emanuel LL. The economics of dying. The illusion of cost savings at the end of life. *New Engl J Med*. 1994;330:540-544.
9. Code of Federal Regulations, Part 418, Medicare Hospice Regulations. 1993.
10. Hadlock DC. Physicians' roles in hospice care. In: Corr CA, Coor DM, eds. *Hospice Care, Principles and Practice*. New York: Springer; 1983:103.

KEY REFERENCES

Articles/Chapters

1. A controlled trial to improve care for seriously ill hospitalized patients. The study to understand prognoses for outcomes and risks of treatments (SUPPORT). The SUPPORT Principal Investigators. *JAMA*. 1995;274:1591-1598.
2. AGS (American Geriatrics Society). Measuring quality of care at the end of life: a statement of principles. *J Am Geriatr Soc*. 1997;45:526-527.
3. Berry ZS, Lynn J. Hospice medicine. *JAMA*. 1993;270:221-223.
4. Billings JA. What is palliative care? *J Palliat Med*. 1998;1:73-81.
5. Billings JA, Block S. Palliative care in undergraduate medical education. Status report and future directions. *JAMA*. 1997;278:733-738.
6. Breitbart W, Bruera E, Chochinov H, Lynch M. Neuropsychiatric syndromes and psychological symptoms in patients with advanced cancer. *J Pain Symptom Manage*. 1995;10:131-141.
7. Breitbart W, Jacobsen PB. Psychiatric symptom management in terminal care. *Clin Geriatr Med*. 1996;12:329-47.
8. Buckman R. Communication in palliative care: a practical guide. In: Doyle D, Hanks GWC, MacDonald N, eds. *Oxford Textbook of Palliative Medicine*, 2nd ed. New York: Oxford University Press; 1996:47-61.
9. Bulkin W, Lukashok H. Rx for dying: the case for hospice. *N Engl J Med*. 1988;318:376-378.
10. Byock I. Hospice and palliative care: a parting of the ways or a path to the future? *J Palliat Med*. 1998;1:165-176.
11. Byock I. When suffering persists. *J Palliat Care*. 1994;10(2):8-13.
12. Byock IR. The nature of suffering and the nature of opportunity at the end of life. *Clin Geriatr Med*. 1996;12(2):237-252.
13. Cassel CK, Vladeck BC. Sounding board. ICD-9 code for palliative or terminal care. *New Engl J Med*. 1996;335:1232-1234.
14. Cassell EJ. The nature of suffering. *New Engl J Med*. 1982;306:639-645.
15. Cherny NI, Coyle N, Foley KM. Suffering in the advanced cancer patient: a definition and taxonomy. *J Palliat Care*. 1994;10:57-70.
16. Cherny NI, Portenoy RK. Sedation in the management of refractory symptoms: guidelines for evaluation and treatment. *J Palliat Care*. 1994;10(2):31-39.
17. Christakis NA. Timing of referral of terminally ill patients to an outpatient hospice. *J Gen Intern Med*. 1994;9(63):14-320.
18. Christakis N, Escarce J. Survival of Medicare patients after enrollment in hospice programs. *N Engl J Med*. 1996; 335:172-8.
19. Cleeland CS, Gonin R, Hatfield AK, et. al. Pain and its treatment in outpatients with metastatic cancer. *N Engl J Med*. 1994;330:592-596.
20. Corr CA, Doka KJ. Current models of death, dying, and bereavement. *Crit Care Nurs Clin North Am*. 1994; 6:545-552.
21. Coyle N, Adelhardt J, Foley KM, Portenoy RK. Character of terminal illness in the advanced cancer patient: pain and other symptoms during the last four weeks of life. *J Pain Symptom Manage*. 1990;5(2):83-93.
22. Donnelly S, Walsh D, Rybicki L. The symptoms of advanced cancer in 1000 patients. *J Palliat Care*. 1994;10:57.
23. Doukas DJ, Gorenflo DW. Analyzing the values history: an evaluation of patient medical values and advance directives. *J Clin Ethics*. 1993;4(1):41-45.
24. Emanuel EJ. Cost savings at the end of life: what do the data show? *JAMA*. 1996:275(24): 1907-1914.

25. Emanuel LL, Emanuel EJ. The medical directive: a new comprehensive advance care document. *JAMA*. 1989;261:3299-3295.

26. Ferrell BA, Bradley LA, Cooney LM, et al. The management of chronic pain in older persons. AGS Panel on Chronic Pain in Older Persons. *J Am Geriatr Society*. 1998;46:635-651

27. Foley KM. Management of cancer pain. In: DeVita VT, Hellman S, Rosenberg SA, eds. *Cancer: Principles and Practice of Oncology*. 4th ed. Philadelphia: Lippincott; 1993:2417-2448.

28. Hill TP. Treating the dying patient: the challenge for medical education. *Arch Intern Med*. 1995;155:1265-1269.

29. Kinzbrunner BM. Hospice: what to do when anti-cancer therapy is no longer appropriate, effective, or desired. *Semin Oncol*. 1994;21:792-798.

30. Levy MH. Pharmacologic treatment of cancer pain. *New Engl J Med*. 1996;335(15):1124-1132.

31. Lynn J. An 88-year old woman facing the end of life. *JAMA*. 1997;277(20):1633-1640.

32. Lynn J. Caring at the end of our lives. *New Engl J Med*. 1996;335(3):201-202.

33. Lynn J, Harrell F, Cohn F, Wagner D, Connors AF. Prognoses of seriously ill hospitalized patients on the days before death: implications for patient care and public policy. *New Horiz*. 1997; 5(1):56-61.

34. MacDonald N. Palliative care: the fourth phase of cancer prevention. *Cancer Detect Prev*. 1991;15:253-255.

35. McCann RM, Hall W, Groth-Junker A. Comfort care for terminally ill patients, the appropriate use of nutrition and hydration. *JAMA*. 1994;272:1263-1266.

36. McCue, J. The naturalness of dying. *JAMA*. 1995;273:1039-1043.

37. Mor V, Kidder D. Cost savings in hospice: final results of the National Hospice Study. *Health Serv Res*. 1985;20:407-422.

38. Mor V, Masterson-Allen S. A comparison of hospice vs. conventional care of the terminally ill cancer patient. *Oncology (Huntingt)*. 1990;4:85-91.

39. Morrison RS, Meier DE, Calles CK. When too much is too little. *New Engl J Med*. 1996;335(23):1755-1759.

40. Parkes CM. Bereavement. In: Doyle D, Hanks GWC, MacDonald N, eds. *Oxford Textbook of Palliative Medicine*. New York: Oxford University Press; 1993:665-678.

41. Portenoy RK. Opioid therapy for chronic nonmalignant pain: a review of the critical issues. *J Pain Symptom Manage*. 1996;11(4):203-217.

42. Rhymes J. Hospice care in America. *JAMA*. 1990;264:369-372.

43. Schonwetter R, Robinson BE. Educational objectives for medical training in the care of the terminally ill. *Acad Med*. 1994;69(8):688-690.

44. Storey P, Hill HH, St. Louis RH, Tarver EE. Subcutaneous infusions for control of cancer symptoms. *J Pain Symptom Manage*. 1990;5:33-41.

45. Teno JM, Lynn J, Connors AF, et al. The illusion of end-of-life resource savings with advance directives. *J Am Geriatr Soc*. 1997;45:513-518.

46. Ventafridda, et. al. Symptom prevalence and control during cancer patients' last days of life. *J Palliat Care*. 1990;6:7-11.

47. vonGunten C, Martinez J. AIDS and palliative medicine: medical treatment issues. *J Palliat Care*. 1995;11(2):5-9.

48. Walsh D. Palliative care: management of the patient with advanced cancer. *Semin Oncol*. 1994;21(suppl 7):100-106.

49. Weissman DE. Pre-clinical palliative medicine education at the Medical College of Wisconsin. *J Cancer Educ*. 1993;8:191-195.

50. Weissman DE. Consultation in palliative medicine. *Arch Intern Med*. 1997;157:733-737.

Books

1. Appleton M, Henschell T. *At Home with Terminal Illness: A Family Guide to Hospice in the Home.* Englewood Cliffs, NJ: Prentice Hall Career & Technology; 1995.
2. Armstrong DA, Goltzer SZ. *Hospice Care for Children.* New York: Oxford University Press; 1993.
3. Buckman R. *How to Break Bad News: A Guide for Health Care Professionals.* Baltimore, Md: The Johns Hopkins University Press; 1992.
4. Bruera E, Portenoy RK, eds. *Topics in Palliative Care Volume 2.* New York: Oxford University Press; 1998.
5. Byock IR. *Dying Well: The Prospect for Growth at the End of Life.* New York: Riverhead Books; 1997.
6. Cassell EJ. *The Nature of Suffering and the Goals of Medicine.* New York: Oxford University Press; 1991.
7. Doyle D, Hanks GWC, MacDonald N, eds. *Oxford Textbook of Palliative Medicine.* New York: Oxford University Press; 1993.
8. Doyle D, Hanks GWC, MacDonald N, eds. *Oxford Textbook of Palliative Medicine.* 2nd ed. New York: Oxford University Press; 1996.
9. Dunlop R. *Cancer: Palliative Care.* London: Springer-Verlag London Limited; 1998.
10. Faulkner A, Maguire P. *Talking to Cancer Patients and Their Relatives.* New York: Oxford University Press; 1994.
11. Field MJ, Cassel CK, eds. *Approaching Death: Improving Care at the End of Life.* Report by the Committee on Care at the End of Life. Institute of Medicine. Washington, D.C.: National Academy Press; 1997.
12. Garrett TM, Baillie HW, Garrett RM. *Health Care Ethics: Principles and Problems.* Englewood Cliffs, NJ: Prentice Hall; 1993.
13. Higginson I, ed. *Clinical Audit in Palliative Care.* New York: Radcliffe Medical Press; 1993.
14. Holland JC, Rowland JH, eds. *Handbook of Psycho-oncology: Psychological Care of the Patient with Cancer.* New York: Oxford University Press; 1990.
15. Hoskin P, Makin W. *Oncology for Palliative Medicine.* New York: Oxford University Press; 1998.
16. Lerman D, Tehan C. *Hospital-Hospice Management Models: Integration and Collaboration.* Chicago, Ill: American Hospital Publishing; 1995.
17. MacDonald N, ed. *Palliative Medicine: A Case-Based Manual.* New York: Oxford University Press; 1998.
18. Mor V, Greer D, Kastenbaum R, eds. *The Hospice Experiment.* Baltimore, Md: The John Hopkins University Press; 1989.
19. Portenoy RK. *Pain in Oncologic and AIDS Patients.* Newtown, Pa: Handbooks in Health Care; 1998.
20. Portenoy RK, Bruera E, eds. *Topics in Palliative Care, Volume 1.* New York: Oxford University Press; 1997.
21. Randall F, Downie RS. *Palliative Care Ethics: A Good Companion.* New York: Oxford Medical Publications, Oxford University Press; 1996.
22. Ray MC. *I'm Here to Help: A Hospice Worker's Guide to Communicating with Dying People and Their Loved Ones.* Mound, Minn: Hospice Handouts, McRay Company; 1992.
23. Saunders C, Kastenbaum R, eds. *Hospice Care on the International Scene.* New York: Springer Publishing Company; 1997.
24. Schonwetter, RS, ed. *Clinics in Geriatric Medicine. Care of the Terminally Ill Patient.* Philadelphia: WB Saunders; 1996:12(2):237-433.
25. Twycross R. *Introducing Palliative Care.* New York: Radcliffe Medical Press; 1997.
26. Twycross R. *Symptom Management in Advanced Cancer.* Abington, Oxon, United Kingdom: Radcliffe Medical Press; 1997.
27. Waller A, Caroline N. *Handbook of Palliative Care in Cancer.* Newton, Mass: Butterworth-Heinemann; 1996.
28. Woodruff R. *Palliative Medicine,* 2nd ed. Melbourne: Asperula Pty Ltd; 1996.
29. Woodruff R. *Palliative Medicine: Symptomatic and Supportive Care for Patients with Advanced Cancer and AIDS.* Victoria, Australia: Asperula Pty Ltd; 1993.

Journals

1. Hospice Journal
   10 Alice Street
   Binghamton, New York 13904-1580
   Telephone: 800/429-6784
   Fax: 800/895-0582

2. Journal of Palliative Care
   Center for Bioethics
   Clinical Research Institute of Montreal
   110 PineAvenue W.
   Montreal, Quebec, Canada H2W 1R7

3. Journal of Pain and Symptom Management
   Elsevier Science, Inc.
   655 Avenue of the Americas
   New York, New York 10010
   Telephone: 212/633-3730
   Fax: 212/633-3680

4. Journal of Palliative Medicine
   Mary Ann Liebert, Inc.
   2 Madison Ave
   Larchmont, NY 10538
   Telephone: 800/M-Liebert
   e-mail: info@liebertpub.com

5. Palliative Medicine
   Arnold Hodder Headline PLC
   London, England, United Kingdom
   Telephone: 44 (0) 1462 672 555
   Fax: 44 (0) 1462 480 947

Other Publications

1. American Pain Society Quality of Care Committee. Quality Improvement Guidelines for the Treatment of Acute Pain and Cancer Pain. *JAMA*. 1995;274(23):1874-1880.
2. *Cancer Pain Relief and Palliative Care: Report of a WHO Expert Committee*. Geneva, Switzerland: World Health Organization Technical Report Series, 804. 1990.
3. *Caring for the Dying: Identification and Promotion of Physician Competency*. Philadelphia, Pa: American Board of Internal Medicine: 1996. Educational Resource Document.
4. *Caring for the Dying: Identification and Promotion of Physician Competency. Personal Narratives*. Philadelphia, Pa: American Board of Internal Medicine: 1996.
5. Centers for Disease Control and Prevention. USPHS/IDSA guidelines for the prevention of opportunistic infections in persons infected with HIV: a summary. *MMWR*. 1995;44(RR-8):1-34.
6. Houts PS, ed. *Home Care Guide for Advanced Cancer: When Quality of Life is the Primary Goal of Care*. Philadelphia, Pa: American College of Physicians: 1995.
7. Jacox A, Carr DB, Payne R, et. al. *Management of Cancer Pain—Clinical Practice Guideline, No. 9*. AHCPH Publication No. 94-0592. Rockville, Md. Agency for Health Care Policy and Research, U.S. Department of Health and Human Services, Public Health Service, March 1994.
8. Johanson GA. *Physicians Handbook of Symptom Relief in Terminal Care*, 4th ed. Santa Rosa, Calif: Sonoma County Academic Foundation for Excellence in Medicine; 1994.
9. Palmetto Government Benefits Administrators: Medicare Advisory Hospice 97-11. Hospice provisions enacted by the Balanced Budget Act (BBA) of 1997. September, 1997.
10. *Pathways for Facing Terminal Illness*. Arlington, Va: National Hospice Organization; 1997.
11. Precepts of palliative care. Robert Wood Johnson National Policy Statements in End-of-Life Care. *J Palliat Med*. 1998;1(2):109-113.
12. Standards and Accreditation Committee: Medical Guidelines Task Force of the National Hospice Organization. *Medical Guidelines for Determining Prognosis in Selected Non-Cancer Diseases*, 2nd Edition. Arlington, Va: National Hospice Organization; 1996.
13. *Standards of a Hospice Program of Care*. Arlington, Va: National Hospice Organization; 1993.
14. Storey P, Knight CF. *UNIPAC One: The Hospice/Palliative Medicine Approach to End-of-Life Care*. American Academy of Hospice and Palliative Medicine. Dubuque, Iowa: Kendall/Hunt Publishing Company; 1998.

15. Storey P, Knight CF. *UNIPAC Two: Alleviating Psychological and Spiritual Pain in the Terminally Ill.* American Academy of Hospice and Palliative Medicine. Dubuque, Iowa: Kendall/Hunt Publishing Company; 1997.
16. Storey P, Knight CF. *UNIPAC Three: Assessment and Treatment of Pain in the Terminally Ill.* Academy of Hospice and Palliative Medicine. Dubuque, Iowa: Kendall/Hunt Publishing Company; 1996.
17. Storey P, Knight CF. *UNIPAC Four: Management of Selected Nonpain Symptoms in the Terminally Ill.* American Academy of Hospice and Palliative Medicine. Dubuque, Iowa: Kendall/Hunt Publishing Company; 1996.
18. Storey P, Knight CF. *UNIPAC Five: Caring for the Terminally Ill: Communication and the Physician's Role on the Interdisciplinary Team.* American Academy of Hospice and Palliative Medicine. Dubuque, Iowa: Kendall/Hunt Publishing Company; 1998.
19. Storey P, Knight CF. *UNIPAC Six: Ethical and Legal Decision Making When Caring for the Terminally Ill.* American Academy of Hospice and Palliative Medicine. Dubuque, Iowa: Kendall/Hunt Publishing Company; 1996.

INDEX

Physician involvement, dying process, 162-163
Physiological changes, dying process, 159-160
Pilocarpine, 85
Plicamycin, 60
Pneumocystis carinii pneumonia (PCP), 120
Pneumonia, 78
Polydipsia, 59
Polyuria, 59
Post-herpetic neuralgia, 122
Post-herpetic neuropathy, 45
Post-limb amputation, 45
Postmastectomy pain, 45
Postnephrectomy pain, 45
Post-radical neck dissection pain, 45
Postthoracotomy pain, 45
Prayer, and stress, 28
Prednisone, 67
Pressure sores, 71-72
Primary afferent fibers, 34
Primary central nervous system lymphoma (PCNSL), 122
Prochlorperazine, 53
Progestins, 67
Prognosis, non-cancer illnesses, 129-130
Projection neuron, 37
Prokinetic drugs, 67
Propofol, 79
Prostaglandins, 34-35
Prostate, 95
Prostatitis, 94
Pruritus, 70-71
Pseudohematuria, 95
Psychosocial aspects, 137-144
    beliefs, 138
    bereavement, 139-140
    conflict, 138
    culture, 138-139
    existential concerns, 139
    grief, 139-140
    impairment, 138
    independence, 139
    interventions, 139
    past experiences, 138
    quality of life, 140-141
    role function, 138
    sexuality, 139
    spiritual concerns, 139
    suffering, 137-138
Psychosocial issues, HIV, 124
Psychosocial modalites, for pain control, 55
Psychostimulants, 54
Psychotherapy, 55
Pulmonary emboli, 77, 79
Pulsus paradoxicus, 61
Pyelography, 95
Pyelonephritis, 93

Q

Quality Assurance, 20
Quality of life (QOL), 7, 140-141

R

Radiation induced neuropathy, 45
Radiation therapy, 77
Rapid escalation of pain, 64
Recertification, medical director and, 18
References, key, 175-179
    articles, 175-176
    books, 177
    chapters, 175-176
    journals, 178
    other, 178-179
Reimbursement mechanisms, 167-171
    HIV, 124
    pediatrics, 111
Relaxation, 55
Renal colic, 93
Renal function, and opioids, 53
Research, and medical director, 21
Routes of drug delivery, 54
    buccal, 54
    rectal, 54
    sublingual, 54
    transdermal, 54
    vaginal, 54

S

Scopolamine patches, 79
Scrotal pain, 94
Secretions, respiratory, 79
Sedatives, 70
Seizures, 63-64, 103-104
Selective serotonin reuptake inhibitors (SSRI), 102, 122
Self-loathing, 140
Sensitization, defined, 33
Serotonin, 34, 37
Serum calcium level, 59-60
Sexuality, 139
Side effects of NSAIDs, 52
Sleep disturbances, 70
Slippery slope, and PAS, 156
Somatic pain, 33
Somatosensory cortex, 36
Somatostatin, 34
Spinal cord compression, 60-61
Spinothalamic tract, 35
Spiritual aspects, 145-151
    of communication, 26
    growth, end of life, 147-148

and HIV, 124
    impact on physicians, 148
    indicators of suffering, 145-146
    interventions, 147
    physician's role in, 146-147
    psychosocial, 139
Standards of care, 10-11
    interdisciplinary team, 10-11
    role of programs, 10
    unit of care, 10
Status epilepticus, defined, 103
Steroids, 77, 79. *See also* Corticosteroids
Stomatitis, 85
Stress management techniques, 28
Substance P, 34, 35
Suffering, 137-138
    indicators of, 145-146
    interventions, 139
    multidimensional nature of, 145
Suicide, 102
Superior vena cava obstruction, 61
SUPPORT study, 129
Surgery, spinal cord compression and, 60
Symptom relief, dying process, 160-162
Symptoms. *See* Non-pain, general

T

Tachycardia, 61
Taste, altered, 86
Tax Equity and Fiscal Responsibility Act (TEFRA), 9
Teaching methods, 3-4
Team education, and medical director, 19
Team physician, 21
Terminal restlessness, 70
Terminally ill, defined, 10
Thalamus, 36
Thoracic aortic dissection, 80
Thrombocytopenia, 63
Thromboxanes, 34
Tietze's syndrome, 80
Total pain assessment, 42
Total parenteral nutrition (TPN), 68
Transcutaneous electrical nerve stimulation (TENS), 55
Transduction of pain, 34-35
Transmission of pain, 35-36
Tricyclic antidepressants (TCA) , 37-38, 122
Tumor infiltration of nerve, 45
Tumor invasion, liver parenchyma and, 89
Tumor necrosis factor (TNF) , 67

U

Ulcerating tumors, 71
Uremia, 67
Ureter, 95
Ureteral pain, 93-95
Urinary obstruction, 62. *See also*
    Genitourinary symptoms
Utilization review, medical director
    and, 20

V

Vasoactive intestinal polypeptide
    (VIP), 34-35
Ventroposterolateral nuclei, 36
Ventroposteromedial nuclei, 36
Virtue-based ethics, 156
Visceral pain, 33
Visual analog scale (VAS), 44
Vital capacity, aging and, 51
Vomiting. *See* Nausea

W

World Health Organization, 2, 7, 52

X

Xerostomia, 85